A Way of Working

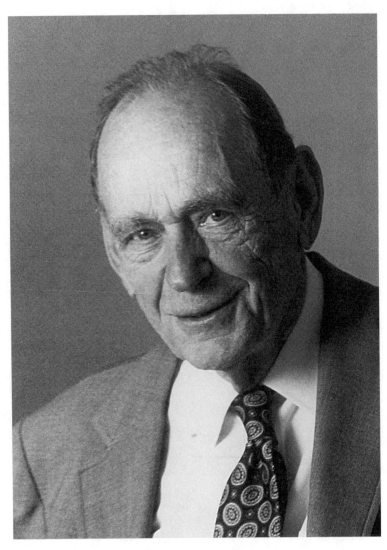

Eugene A. Stead, Jr.

A Way of Working

Essays on the Practice of Medicine

By

Eugene A. Stead, Jr., M.D.

Florence McAlister Emeritus Professor of Medicine
Emeritus Chair of Medicine
Duke University School of Medicine

Edited by

Barton F. Haynes, M.D.

Frederic M. Hanes Professor and Chair
Department of Medicine
Duke University School of Medicine

Carolina Academic Press
Durham, North Carolina

ISBN 0-89089-242-3
LCCN 00-111319

Grateful acknowledgment is made to the following publishers, editors, or authors for permission to reproduce previously published work: North Carolina Medical Journal, Carolina Academic Press, American Medical Association, Archives of Pediatric & Adolescent Medicine (formerly American Journal of Diseases of Children), Annals of Internal Medicine, American College of Physicians-American Society of Internal Medicine, Archives of Internal Medicine, *The Pharos*, Alpha Omega Alpha Honor Medical Society, Academic Medicine-AAMC (formerly Journal of Medical Education), Association of American Medical Colleges, Journal of Medical Systems, Plenum Publishing Co., Bulletin of New York Academic Medicine, Oxford University Press, New England Journal of Medicine, Publishing Division of the Massachusetts Medical Society, Transactions of the Association of American Physicians, The Association of American Physicians, MD Computing, Springer-Verlag Publishing Co., American Journal of Medicine, Journal of American Geriatric Society, Blackwell Science, Inc., Dr. Eugene A. Stead, Jr., and *Resident and Staff Physician, Romaine Pierson Publishers, Inc.* for material that appeared in *Medical Times*.

Carolina Academic Press
700 Kent Street
Durham, North Carolina 27701
Telephone (919) 489-7486
Facsimile (919) 493-5668
E-mail: cap@cap-press.com
www.cap-press.com

Printed in the United States of America.

Dedication

At the end of the day, the practice of medicine is a service occupation, not a license to wealth or social standing. This book is dedicated to those physicians who recognize that it is very difficult to truly be a good doctor, and who derive joy from the hard work of serving others.

Barton F. Haynes, MD
Eugene A Stead, Jr., MD
2001

Contents

II. Academic Medical Centers

III. The Computerized Medical Database: The Way of the Future

IV. The Community and Their Doctors

Contents

Acknowledgments

Many individuals have helped to put together this collection of Eugene A. Stead, Jr. essays. Bess Cebe, Dr. Stead's long-time secretary, worked to support the effort and found unpublished manuscripts from the Stead files. Evelyn Stead and Penny Hodgson provided important editorial assistance and Kim McClammy typed the manuscript. I am grateful to Stan and Doris Tanger for their support of this book project, and for their making the book available to all Duke house staff and medical students. My wife Caroline and my three children Charlotte, Ben, and Laura continue to be loving and patient with all my varied projects. Finally, I am grateful to Dr. Stead for providing unpublished essays and photographs as well as for his mentorship.

Barton F. Haynes, M.D.
Durham, North Carolina
December 2000

Introduction

This is a book of essays written by one of the great doctors of the mid-20th century, Eugene A. Stead, Jr. Gene Stead served in many jobs at Harvard, Cincinnati, Emory and Duke Medical Schools, including Chair of Medicine at Emory and Duke, but I will let Dr. Stead introduce you to himself in the *Prologue: Eugene Stead on Eugene Stead*. Gene Stead's contributions to American Medicine are in two general areas: his effect on the doctor-patient relationship that is written about in a companion volume, "A Way of Thinking" by Dr. Eugene A. Stead, Jr., and his effect on healthcare systems in the U.S. that is written about in this volume "A Way of Working."

In this volume, essays and papers are collected that reflect Stead's impact on various systems in American medicine, such as training programs, academic health centers, national organizations, and the formation of a new profession: the physician's assistant. These essays show the extraordinary vision he has had over the years to anticipate the future.

The chapters in the first section "Medical Education For the Future," reflect Stead's vision on medical students and housestaff training and review his pioneering work in changing the Duke curriculum. His success in training young doctors is indicated by the 33 Stead trainees who went on to become chairs of medicine.

In the section "Academic Medical Centers," Stead gives out his secrets for administering departments and medical centers— secrets that are as relevant today as they were in years past. These sections are a "must read" for contemporary chairs of medicine and their deans. In addition, he anticipated the crisis today in nursing and other health provider shortages and proposed a series of innovative ways to bring healthcare teams together.

In the section on computerized medical databases, Stead shows us his vision in foretelling the future by telling us in the 1970s of the importance of computers in medicine today. Thirty years ago Stead started the Duke cardiovascular database that now has clinical data on over 250,000 patients. Papers written out of the database have changed the way cardiovascular medicine is practiced today in the U.S. Most importantly, the Duke Clinical Research Institute (led by Stead protégé, Dr. Robert Califf) grew out of the Department of Medicine Cardiology Database, and now is a force in clinical research internationally, not only for cardiovascular medicine, but also for minority health, neurobiology, and other disciplines as well.

In the section on the medical workforce, Stead's classic papers on his establishment of the physician–assistant profession are reprinted, and chronicle the development of his greatest innovation and most successful program.

Finally, in the section on healthcare and the nation, Stead addresses many of the unsolved social problems that we still face, such as poverty and lack of healthcare for all citizens in the US, and proposes several solutions to these social ills.

It is remarkable how many trends, events and medical advances Gene Stead has anticipated and predicted over the years: computer databases in medicine, evidence-based medicine, modern medical school curricula, the effects of managed care on academic health center research and teaching, the nursing shortage, the success of the physician's assistant program, and the importance of genetics and genetic screening in preventive medicine. Because of his ability to see the future, the words that Gene Stead has written over the past 50 years are just as relevant today as when they were written. His essays are packed with wisdom, wit, and perspective, and his story is told in a straightforward voice that is uniquely his.

Barton F. Haynes, M.D.
Durham, North Carolina
December 2000

Prologue

Eugene Stead on Eugene Stead

Eugene Stead Jr. is a 92-year-old Georgia boy educated at Emory College and Emory Medical School. His apprenticeships included medical and surgical internships at the Peter Bent Brigham Hospital, a tour of duty at the Cincinnati General Hospital, a two year stint as chief resident at the Thorndike Memorial Hospital located on the grounds of the Boston City Hospital, and a two year term on the junior faculty of Harvard Medical School. He was appointed Professor of Medicine and Chairman of the Department at Emory at the age of 33. He spent the years of World Ward II at Grady Hospital where he operated the medical service with 3rd and 4th year medical students. From Friday through Sunday he lived at Grady studying circulatory failure from knife, ice-pick and gun wounds. When trauma patients were not available, he and his colleagues studied patients with heart failure. They were always present.

In 1945, Stead was made Dean of Emory Medical School. He was an example of the Peter Principle. He had been promoted to his level of incompetence. He licked the Peter Principle by resigning as Dean and returned to a level of his competence. January 1, 1949 he became Professor and Chairman of the Department of Medicine at Duke.

He resigned his position as chairman at the age of 60. After surveying the field he found no example of a chairman, 60 years or older, who was as productive as Stead had been between 33

xv

and 60. The odds were great that after the age of 60 his department would slowly lose some of its excellence.

He is still active at the age of 92. He has had an unusual opportunity to observe students from their second year in medical school to their maturation as doctors, scientists and educators.

Through these years of activity he has evolved many general precepts. Some of them are:

1) Students do the learning and they should have the honors;

2) Selection of the people who are admitted to a program is much more important than the course of study. Input largely determines output;

3) The faculty fiddles with the curriculum but activity of the student is only affected by examinations. Examinations test memory and until examinations become open book, medical students will continue to memorize useless facts;

4) Examinations have to emphasize useless facts because you can not arrange a string of students from top to bottom if you only ask for useful facts;

5) Physician associates and assistants can increase the productivity of doctors without impairing the quality of health care;

6) The sign of each experience is more important than the facts memorized. If the sign is negative, students will shun the area. If the sign is positive, they may continue to explore and learn;

7) Never give assignments. Identify areas that are of interest and see how far students will go on their own;

8) Many persons with excellent grades and high IQs will sit on their bottoms. The work of the world is

done by those who get up in the morning, enjoy the day and make little distinction between work and play;

9) Don't forget the forgetting curve. Ask questions over the years to discover what is best left in books and computers;

10) Any form of active learning will accumulate fewer facts per hour but will slow the forgetting curve;

11) Education is never efficient;

12) Any question to which there is a known answer can be reduced to memory. The best questions have no absolute answers; and

13) Availability is a more useful attribute than brilliance. People who are happy stay home — the discontented travel.

A Way of Working

I

Medical Education for the Future

The care of the patients should be carried out by doctors who are interested in giving service to people. Good doctors believe that patients can legitimately make demands on doctors, and because the ill are not rational, these demands do not have to be rational.

Chapter 1
Origin of the Species

M edical schools have tight control over medical manpower.[1] They determine the number of persons entering the profession, and they determine the cultural mix of the profession. Such great power can be tolerated only when it is used with wisdom and discretion to meet the broad needs of society.

In winter of 1962, the suggestion was made by some of our scientists that calculus be made a mandatory requirement for admission to medical school. I thought then and do now that the needs of the country for doctors cannot be met by arbitrary, fixed requirements forcing all doctors to become more and more alike. I recorded my thoughts as follows.

I do believe that the opportunities in biology for the student with abilities in mathematics, chemistry and physics are greater than they have ever been, even though many of the premedical advisors still believe that the traditional medical school curriculum prepares students both for practice and research. In the last twenty years medical schools have become an excellent place for training and research in biology. The average premedical advisor still thinks of a medical school as a place to train a doctor who will care for patients. He is well aware that the doctor in practice never uses mathematics, chemistry, physics or the information

---

1. Stead EA, Jr. Origin of the species. *Medical Times*, 98:223-224, 1970.

science, and he tends to advise students with these abilities to enter the physical sciences. I would like the premedical advisors to be better aware of the fact that most medical schools now produce biological scientists whose range of competencies go far beyond that of those needed for the care of patients. These scientists will not care for many sick patients.

Before the start of World War II in 1939, practicing doctors talked only to other practicing doctors. There were only a few research programs where doctors talked to persons skilled in the wide variety of scientific disciplines which now underlie the medical enterprise. After the war, the role of the National Institutes of Health increased rapidly both in facilities for in-house research and in financial support of medical schools who could bring in a variety of non-medical scientists to support the medical enterprise.

Most medical educators are conscious of the great changes that tax supported research funds made in the composition of medical school faculties. Schools with a diverse faculty from the wide range of disciplines that now supported the medical enterprise were quickly funded and doctors now talked to scientists who had never before influenced the practice of medicine. There is a tendency to credit the rapid changes in the composition of medical faculties and the great strides made in patient care to the grant supported programs of the NIH. I believe that the in-house NIH programs were the more important. The changes in the universities were slow because there was no large pool of more widely trained scientific doctors to staff a large number of residents. The NIH programs were already staffed with scientists and young doctors were engaged in all NIH activities. The military wisely decided to defer doctors who were given NIH appointments to work in a wide array of scientific disciplines. Those appointments particularly in the areas of cardiology, endocrinology, and metabolic diseases, where links of the new biological supported sciences to new treatments of diseases were most obvious, became very competitive. The most desirable NIH posts went to graduates of Harvard, major medical schools in New York, Chicago, Hopkins, Philadelphia and Washington University.

How could upcoming schools like Emory and Duke compete with better established schools? We had one thing on our side. The number of most favored places was limited and most of the best prepared undergraduate and graduate students only applied for the most desirable positions. I looked the situation over and saw that the personnel of all the in-house Institutes were very similar. They were all trying to broaden their understanding of biology by bringing in the wide variety of disciplines not commonly very important in the education of practicing doctors. The scientist and the laboratories of scientists in the Dental Institute were remarkably similar to those in the Heart Institute. A doctor with a traditional medical school education (Emory and Duke students) had for the first time to work with and talk to other scientists who had never cared for a patient and had no intention of practicing medicine.

We urged our bright folks to apply to the less popular positions and in term of absolute numbers of NIH appointments from our supposedly weak school came out very well. Since our graduates preformed beyond the expectation of the NIH our stock went up rapidly and eventually we obtained our share of appointments to the more sought after positions.

In summary I support a less popular position: That the in-house programs of the NIH had a greater effect on the bringing of new sciences into medicine than the awarding of NIH funds to university departments.

The care of the patients will be carried out by doctors who are interested in giving service to people. They will be more interested in the integrative behavior of the organism than in molecular biology. They will have the ability to use the concepts and machines which are created by the scientist but they will have little interest in the component parts of these black boxes. They will learn how to use any tool that is helpful in caring for their patients, but they will not be interested in learning for the sake of learning. This division between the thinkers and doers is related to the number of hours in the working day. The wider the interests and the more aspects of any problems that are examined, the fewer are the patients seen.

Physicians have a large educational role in their work. They are aware that many of their patients have difficulty in reading, some are tone deaf, others have difficulty in word-association. Many of their patients have difficulty in learning in the area of interpersonal relationships, in the area of social relations, in the sexual field or in the political field. These problems in learning are intensified by the presence of any disease process.

Students destined to be medical scientists have been picked for their ability to handle abstract ideas and to perform well in mathematics, chemistry and physics. Because they are well endowed with the necessary equipment to learn in these areas, they need little help. In many other areas of learning they may be extraordinarily inept. They not only will have difficulty in learning from the usual interpersonal and social situations but they will have even greater difficulty in helping other people who are handicapped by difficulties in learning in these same areas.

I would admit into medical school a wide spectrum of students, many quite inept with calculus. I would allow differentiation in medical school to occur between the scientist and the practicing physician. I would train them both in the same school and with the same teachers. The scientist would see less of the clinical service and the "doctor-to-be" less of the basic science area. I would allow free movement back and forth for those students who had the ability to perform well in both areas.

Now as in 1962,[2] these principles still seem sound. I would further broaden the "mix" within the profession by admitting into the medical schools more talent from the fields of engineering, information sciences, business administration and economics. I would require less training in the biosciences for these new categories of students.

Doctors perform too many functions, carry too widely different responsibilities, live too many lives, to be recruited from a narrow segment of our society.

---

2. In 1962, Eugene Stead, Phillip Handler, the Chair of Biochemistry at Duke and others reorganized the Duke Medical School curriculum. All basic science didactic sessions were in Year 1, and clinical clerkships were in Year 2, and the third year was devoted entirely to independent study. The fourth year generally was comprised of clinical electives. The curriculum remains largely the same today, in 2001.

Chapter 2

To Manage or Not To Manage

We have never made a strong effort to recruit into the medical profession students interested in management.[1] The strong bioscience orientation of our early medical education has tended to discourage students with other interests and skills from entering medical school. If such students did enter medical school, they were forced to devote two years to memorizing material that had little relevance to practice but was a hurdle that must be jumped before they could become doctors. The net effect of the system has been to produce few physicians with superior managerial talents.

It can be argued that in this day of specialization doctors should practice medicine and leave the management of the health area to non-physicians. This is certainly the current trend. But the non-doctor is always at a disadvantage because he does not understand the problems of either the patients or the professionals. Before I burn all my bridges behind me and accept non-physician management as the best solution, I should like to try to field teams of capable doctor-managers.

No academic area has been outstanding in attracting talent to the field of medical administration. The public health schools do not, generally, have student bodies of outstanding abilities. The

---

1. Stead EA, Jr. To manage or not to manage. *Medical Times*, 97:241-242, 1969.

schools of hospital administration are a dull bunch. William Anlyan[2] is an exception. I believe that the medical schools have the potential of drawing the best talent.

If we are to produce doctor-managers who are knowledgeable in political science, law, economics, information transfer and systems engineering, students must be sought in academic areas other than the bioscience divisions. We must catch the interest of undergraduate students who would normally seek a career via one of the more progressive schools of business administration. This recruitment can succeed only if schools of medicine allow disciplines other than the traditional biosciences to serve the purpose of teaching the budding doctor to think, to learn symbolic languages and to solve problems. These students would then be taught only that amount of bioscience that is tightly coupled to medicine. Doctors trained in this way would be as able practitioners as our present product. Practice, administration and biomedical research are the three common paths doctors travel. Students trained with less investment in bioscience would have the paths of practice and administration open to them; they would find the bioscience research path, for practical purposes, closed.

Theoretically, many medical schools already accept students with widely different educational backgrounds. In fact, they have required each student, regardless of his or her background, to jump the same bioscience hurdle in medical school. This has kept most bright students with limited bioscience backgrounds out of medical school. Those who dared the cold water had to make a tremendous investment in memorizing over a four-year period. By the end of that time their original potential assets had been lost.

---

2. William G. Anlyan, M.D. is the former Dean of Duke Medical School, 1964 to 1988.

The time has come for medical schools to admit a wider spectrum of students and to put out a more diverse product.[3]

---

3. This essay, written in 1969, has largely been adapted by Duke and other medical schools. At Duke, medical students can now pursue MD–MPH, MD–MBA, and MD–master's in public policy combined programs.

Chapter 3

Intern and Residency Training

E ach of us doctors is the product of a medical school, and most of us have taken intern and residency training.[1] Medical schools and hospitals are undergoing rapid changes in structure and function, and from time to time we need to be made aware of the changes.

The majority of medical students, before applying for postgraduate appointments, have begun to visit hospitals for a first hand look at intern and residency programs. Hundreds of students are interviewed by hundreds of faculty members each year. What goes on behind those closed doors? Let me open my door and give you my pitch.

What schools should the senior visit? In my senior year, I was impressed by three young doctors who were interested in students and spent a considerable amount of time caring for patients in our city hospital. They learned new things every day and shared their experiences with the students and the resident staff. I knew that I wanted to become a caring doctor and enjoy a life-time of learning. My three role models suggested that I apply to Presbyterian Hospital in New York and three hospitals in Boston, the Peter Bent Brigham, the Harvard Services at the

---

1. Stead EA, Jr. Intern and residency training. *Medical Times*, 94:1001–1004, 1966.

Boston City Hospital, and the Massachusetts General Hospital. They identified the professors of medicine at each hospital and suggested that I go to the library and read the papers that they were publishing in current medical journals. These hospitals required applicants to visit their hospital and have interviews with several senior professors. The applicants had the chance to talk with interns and residents and determine if these institutions were producing a product that they admired. My first choice was Peter Bent Brigham and I spent 2½ happy years there.

The training of physicians is the purpose of the Department of Medicine at Duke University. Experience has taught us that the selection of the internship is the most important decision of a physician's professional life. This experience will mold young doctors more than any other. As you examine prospective programs, you pay primary attention to product. Do they have the capacity and desire to grow the kind of person that you want to become? Duke is not for everybody, and medicine is a demanding master. Experience has shown that Duke does give a very rewarding experience to intelligent graduates who wish to achieve excellence in medicine.

To accomplish this our staff (1) takes care of patients: sick and well, poor and rich, educated and uneducated; (2) engages in research at many levels; and (3) teaches a wide variety of students. Our prime product is not the care of patients at Duke or the production of new knowledge by research. Young physicians are our prime product—to care for sick and well patients; to do medical research; and to carry out the varied functions needed by the health field. Responsibility for patient care, participation in the teaching program, and close contact with a staff engaged in patient care, research and writing are the essential ingredients for a program charged with producing trained manpower.

The medical internship and residency program at Duke is designed to give the intern a knowledge of the factual material in the field of medicine and a sound philosophical basis for a lifetime of learning in practice. What is done is important, but why it is done is even more important. Duke is not just a collection of excellent doctors. It is a group of doctors who have carefully thought out a program of training that will allow maximum growth of people. The staff does believe that doctors exist to care for people. It does believe that patients can legitimately make demands on doctors and that, because the ill are not rational, these demands do not have to be rational. The staff does believe that the practice of medicine has many emotional and intellectual rewards. It believes that the intellectual rewards of practice can be combined with economic rewards if the physician has learned to care for private patients in a teaching atmosphere.[2] Research and private care can be carried on simultaneously if opportunities have been available for this kind of learning during the training period. The staff believes that there are many pitfalls in learning in the multivariable, ill-characterized systems typified by the patient. The doctor-to-be should have cared for patients of all types; charity patients of several races with no other system of support. Private patients can reject the doctor and go elsewhere. Veterans, middle-class patients, rich patients, cooperative and uncooperative patients, hostile patients, mentally disturbed people; the wider the mix, the better for the doctor-to-be. We have a single faculty to care for the wide mix of patients. The third and fourth year students, the intern and the first-year resident form a close working unit for purposes of learning how to care for patients and for learning how to learn in a system as complex as the patient. Everyone in this unit is both a teacher and a learner. Learning is an active process and

2. "Public" and "Private" wards are now a thing of the past at Duke and most other hospitals, and have given way to private hospital rooms and similar clinics for all patients.

each of us learns more when we teach than when we are being taught.

Some of our interns who come from other schools are surprised at the emphasis we place on the fact that they must teach. They say that since more of our interns will practice than will remain in the university, this emphasis may be misplaced. We take the opposite point of view. The practitioner does more teaching than the academician. The physician-in-practice teaches his office personnel, his paramedical assistants and, above all, his patients. The noise in the information transfer systems, the twist given to one word which inverts the meaning of the whole concept, the differences in the intake systems of two different persons, these are the same whether the intern is trying to teach the student, or the doctor is trying to teach a diabetic patient to live with his disease.

The intern year is a year of doing. Interns must handle a volume of work great enough to make them become efficient in giving medical care. The volume of work must be great enough to make them effective practitioners. They cannot solve their problems by devoting an equal amount of time to each area of the examination. They must explore and rapidly discard the irrelevant areas, but spend as much time as need be on the relevant areas. They will make errors. The staff will pick up these errors and protect the patient from harm. The next time around, the intern will make the right decision.

The intern, as the doer, must be fed intellectually by the student below and by his first-year resident above. By the end of the year they will be comfortable with any patient with any illness. All the rest of their lives they will give patient care quickly and efficiently. Each day, their intern training will give them time for other ventures. The intern year requires a large investment of time and efforts, but it guarantees continued dividends.

The third and fourth years of medical school, the internship, and first year of residency are devoted to teaching the doctor how to care for and to understand people—sick and well. At the end of this time, young doctors appreciate the complexity of the problems in clinical medicine; they understand how to set up learning situations as they care for patients; and they understand the integrated behavior of the organism in which disease processes may occur. Under the guidance of the clinical staff, they have re-read their physiology, pathology, biochemistry, pharmacology, anatomy and microbiology. They have made the connections in their brain between clinical and pre-clinical learning. They are now ready to learn more about the special procedures that are useful in medicine. If they wish to specialize, they may carry this out in many ways. They may spend several years working with specialists in the area of their special competence. They may spend a year rotating through several specialties. They may go to the laboratory to master some of the areas of science that underlie the practice of medicine. They may work out a year of combined clinical and laboratory experiences. There are, then, many ways to use the medical center after the internship and first year residency. We work out specialized programs to fit the diverse needs of our trainees. We try to structure programs to use effectively the years committed to required government service. Productive use of this time is more important than any particular sequence of training.

Chapter 4

Medical Care: Its Social and Organizational Aspects. Postgraduate Medical Education in the Hospital

I nternship and residency years are the golden years in the life of a physician who practices medicine.[1] They are the years when physicians first become professional workers, the years when patients are first willing to entrust their bodies and minds to their care, and the years of close association with bright young colleagues and mature doctors. These are important, formative years, and they shape the future conduct of young physicians more than any other experience. Medical school is important in determining where doctors take their internship and residency. Faculty members, fully conscious of the importance of intern and resident training and with sufficient leisure time to transmit this information to the student, have a larger proportion of their students taking internships and residencies in hospitals where the emphasis is on a program of continuing education. The forces at work during the internship and residency are so strong that, after a short time, the attitudes engendered in the hospital setting become dominant and one cannot identify particular schools on the basis of performance.

1. Stead EA, Jr. Medical Care: Its social and organizational aspects. Postgraduate medical education in the hospital. *N. Eng. J. Med.*, 269:240-244,1961.

When the hospital is owned and administered by a university, the chiefs of the clinical services are in charge of the educational program in their respective areas. As medical educators and clinicians, the chiefs of service can trim the service loads to meet the needs of the educational programs. At the same time, they are in a position to demand that the service functions, accepted as part of the training of interns, are performed well. A university may have a teaching service in a hospital administered by a separate board of trustees. Should the interns and residents be under the administrative control of the university and medical school or under the control of the hospital? The simplest arrangement, the protection of the interests of residents, patients and medical schools, is to give both the medical school and the hospital a hand in the appointment of the chiefs of service. The medical school may have the right of nomination, and the hospital the privilege of accepting or rejecting the nominee. Under these conditions the chiefs of the clinical services have direct responsibility for both education and service, and they in turn are responsible to both the medical school and the hospital.

The goals of the internship and residency must be defined, and the doctors in training must be aware of these goals. Two primary goals may be defined. The first is to teach the doctor in training the best current practice of medicine. Emphasis is placed on common problems and the best immediate solution of them. The second goal is to use the patient's illness for educational purposes, which means that as much time must be spent thinking about what is not known as about what is known. Here, the emphasis is on an understanding of the biologic problems responsible for the behavior of the patient and consideration of what the doctor can do to alter an unfavorable balance between organism and environment. The doctor in training is made ready to read the books that will be written during the next twenty years and is prepared to learn from the scientific meetings of the future. Thus, the internship and residency experience is designed to be quite unlike practice, with the anticipation that much useful knowledge related to practice will be acquired by the physician from his associates during the early years of his practice. All residency programs attempt in part to meet both goals, but commonly, one of the two is emphasized.

The intern and the student should be noncompetitive. The intern moves ahead rapidly and becomes a competent guide for his third-year and fourth-year students. The students can be given considerable responsibility and, during the senior year in medical school, can have many of the experiences normally given to the intern in a rotating service. The fact that interns have elected to spend a full year under the charge of a single department indicates a strong degree of interest in the service, and a great deal of responsibility can safely be given to those interns. They are accepted as an important part of the service and, in a short time, begin to resemble first-year residents more than interns.

Most medical educators would agree that the internship and residency are part of the doctor's educational program and that these years are best spent in a teaching hospital. There are many definitions of a teaching hospital. I have always said that a teaching hospital is one in which the intern and resident can teach, rather than one in which they are taught. Medical students are the greatest single asset of a teaching hospital. Properly woven into the program, they give the intern and resident the opportunity for an active participation in the learning, which can come only from establishing correlations between biologic processes and diseases from the manipulation of ideas and from the painting of word pictures. I know of many ways to teach medical students without the use of interns and residents as teachers. I know of no method of intern and resident training that is as effective as one that involves them directly in the teaching program.

One of the striking developments of the last thirty years has been the appearance of large numbers of people in the university medical centers who are supported by sources other than patient fees. These faculty members are given leisure time to engage in research and teaching. Before this development any physician giving good medical care was as capable of teaching clinical medicine as any member of the university faculty. With the rapid advances in biologic knowledge this situation has changed. Although the university physician and the physician in the community hospital may be equally effective in teaching the medicine of today, the projective aspects will be different. The university faculty member will teach more information pertinent to the medicine of tomorrow.

Many hospitals, not primarily engaged in training, have appreciated the fact that the practicing doctor cannot adequately handle a training program for interns and residents, and they have added one or more full-time doctors to their staffs, either in the role of educational directors or as chiefs of their major services. The success of many of these full-time staff members has been evaluated by the numbers of interns and residents brought into the hospital. In general, these hospitals do not have the depth of university services. There is the inescapable fact that the majority of the staff are primarily interested in practice and not in education. The stimulus of the medical student's presence is usually lacking. Many educational directors are unhappy because professors in medical schools do not recommend that their students take their graduate work in a community hospital. My own observations indicate that those doctors practicing medicine in community hospitals that ask to be supplied with interns advise their own sons and daughters to take their graduate training in a medical center closely tied in with a university and with undergraduate training.

There are many hospitals that lie between the university

medical center and the community hospital. Some are affiliated to a greater or lesser degree with teaching institutions. Many medical schools have appointed the staff of their dean's committee-affiliated Veterans Administration Hospital and have included the Veterans Administration hospital in the university medical center. These units have the necessary faculty for training in depth and for active research programs. Adequate experience with the non-veteran population is achieved by working in both the civilian and Veterans Administration portions of the medical center. Rotation between these two units presents little problem if the services are staffed by a single faculty and the educational program is guided by a common philosophy.

Many excellent clinics, some university affiliated, give excellent training in current medicine. As a group they are less concerned with the projective aspects of the graduate experience. Many of the internships in Army, Navy and Air Force hospitals have excellently planned programs. They miss, however, the stimulus of undergraduate teaching and rarely have the drive of a university medical center staffed by a group of "eager beavers" who work far into the night.

In addition to patient care and teaching, the faculties of most medical centers are heavily involved in research activities. What is the relation of research experience to graduate training? Some services are strongly oriented toward research and give preference to candidates who have engaged in research during their undergraduate years. Some services require one or more years in the laboratory as a part of their program. Others believe that a pattern of critical observation and reading can be developed on the basis of clinical experiences and, if the faculty is research minded, that no formal research training is required. Students take formal research training if they find the experience relevant and if they show some aptitude in the laboratory.

I strongly believe that one should spend the intern and residency years in a setting where the faculty is actively engaged in research. A doctor has the opportunity for two types of learning. One I call "experiential." He or she has lived through a series of experiences with a patient and can describe how the patient behaved, how the family felt and what the doctor did. The situation is so complex and the number of variables so great that the doctor learns nothing that can be applied logically to another patient. Doctors have had an experience that gives them insight into the possibilities inherent in biologic systems, but it has afforded them no understanding of the operation of the system. The second type of learning is that in which the variables are better controlled and specific information that can logically be applied to another patient is gained. Unless these two types of learning are sharply differentiated, a kind of pseudoscience creeps into medicine. Even under the best of circumstances, logic has a limited use in the practice of medicine, because one is always observing the effects of changes in internal or external environment on an undefined substrate. Doctors with curiosity and training in accurate observation will more quickly define the differences in each of their patients than less well-trained doctors. They will develop their curiosity, their ability to make accurate observations and an appreciation of the limitations of prediction in ill-defined systems much more rapidly when their instructors are attempting to establish new knowledge about biologic systems. I do not believe that formal laboratory research training should be given unless the candidate has aptitude and enthusiasm for the venture.

The continued rapid growth of knowledge in the basic sciences has required clinical services to develop programs that will keep interns and residents knowledgeable in these areas. Some services have a highly structured series of basic-science lectures. These are effective if the doctors responsible for patient care know the material presented and have the interns and residents discuss the material as they take care of patients. A few services require that the residents take one year of work in a basic-science department. My own preference is for the unstructured program in which the clinical teachers are familiar with the developments in basic science and demonstrate the usefulness of this knowledge as they care for patients. By appropriate questions they can determine the extent of the resident's knowledge and can arouse interest. They are then in a position to guide the reading of the residents, to refer them to members of the faculty with deeper knowledge in the area, and to listen to residents as they begin to relate their new-found knowledge to patient care.

The number of physicians taking two more years of training in a basic-science department is steadily increasing. Some of this training may be taken in combined M.D.-Ph.D. programs. Other undergraduate students spend equal amounts of time in the basic-science department but do not obtain additional degrees. In many institutions the basic-science work is taken after one or more years of graduate clinical experience. The presence of doctors with basic science experience at both the senior-staff and resident-staff levels makes for good communication between the clinical and preclinical areas. The increasing sophistication of the clinical staff is causing an interesting shift in the teaching assignments of the faculty. The younger clinicians are increasingly urging their basic-science faculties to teach material and concepts that cannot at present be used in clinical practice. They are more interested in the projective aspects of the basic-science years as preparation for the future. The clinicians feel quite competent to teach the aspects of basic science that are presently used in clinical practice. It seems reasonable for this teaching responsibility to be assumed by the clinical faculty in view of the greater number of years spent in clinical training.

Interns and residents are working in clinical services primarily to further their education. They wish to increase their ability to care for sick people and to achieve a firm groundwork so that as they give service for the many years of their practice, they can continue to learn. As advanced students of clinical medicine they, of necessity, perform some service. What should they be paid? The idea of paying them primarily for service has never been seriously proposed for one simple reason: the continued education of the resident and intern requires more funds than the hospital can collect for their services. Even if 100 percent of the income created by the residents were returned to the residents they would still be underpaid.

As advanced students of clinical medicine, they require a faculty and appropriate library and laboratory facilities. They cannot possibly create enough income to pay for the cost of their education. In general, the hospital pays a part of the cost of supplying the clinical laboratory (the hospital), and the university or some other educational agency is largely responsible for the support of the faculty and experimental laboratories. The more money put into the laboratory, the library and the faculty, the less money will be available for scholarships for the clinical graduate students (interns and residents). Just as the excellent university supplied with an outstanding faculty does not suffer for want of students despite a high tuition rate, the excellent clinical service with a good laboratory—that is, a hospital, a fine library, excellent teachers and experimental laboratories—does not suffer for want of graduate students (interns and residents) because its scholarships (intern and resident pay) do not cover the cost of living.

The rate of pay in teaching hospitals is slowly rising. It is being forced up by several factors. The number of students already married at the time of admission to medical school is increasing, and the number of interns and residents with children ready to enter the first grade of school is increasing. These students have exhausted their resources for borrowing before they graduate from medical school, and must be paid at a rate that allows them to accumulate less debt during their graduate years.

Those going into university and governmental positions cannot afford as great a debt at the time of completion of their graduate training as those going into clinical practice. The length of graduate training is greatly prolonged for students who wish to perform in the roles of both scientist and doctor. This increased cost of proficiency in two disciplines cannot be met without some increase in scholarship funds for the graduate years. The standard of living of graduate students in other areas, which receive more adequate scholarship support, is forcing a re-examination of our own practices in the clinical graduate areas.

Should one receive graduate clinical training in the same hospital where one received his undergraduate training? There is no simple answer. From the standpoint of the service it is desirable to have approximately half its graduate students from its own undergraduate service. The faculty has spent many hours in creating the educational climate characteristic of the particular medical center. Students coming from other schools for graduate clinical training need something with a definite identity and purpose. On the other hand, the medical service does not want all its interns or students from its own undergraduate school. It needs both the good advertising it receives when it sends superior students elsewhere and the impact upon itself of superior students from other schools.

The problem for students is more complicated. They may be tied to their undergraduate area by a working spouse, by home ownership or by a good school arrangement for their children. The stronger the medical center, the greater the likelihood that it can serve satisfactorily as both undergraduate and graduate base. The more the medical center is willing to synthesize undergraduate, graduate and service times into a coordinated program, the greater the advantages of not moving. In many medical centers the years spent in basic science departments expose the clinical graduate student to as different a faculty and to as new a philosophy as would be achieved by a much more distant move to the clinical department of another medical center. This adds up to the fact that there are advantages to staying and advantages to moving. Enough students usually decide to stay to meet the needs of the particular services for stability.

One can quickly sense the interest of a specialty area in giving education in depth if one discusses the internship and service time with the chief of the service. If the chief will accept any type of internship and any type of service experience as adequate preparation for his residency program, one should avoid him as one would the plague if one has any real interest in acquiring a background that will prepare one for advancing knowledge. If the chief is interested in the internship and plans with the applicant the use of his service time so that he can bring knowledge to the service that most of the residents do not have, any offer that he makes should be considered most carefully. Many students and interns visit several medical centers. What can they find out? They can discover the general physical surroundings in which they will work. They can examine the products of the service. The senior residents and chief residents are the products that are near the end of the molding. Do the students and interns wish to put forces in play that will make them resemble the products of this medical center? Do residents of this student's character, background and ambition grow in this setting? Is this a program of active learning? Is this a service of such strong traditions that being on it automatically has a favorable effect on one's performance? Are the interns entering the program bright, well motivated and excited about learning clinical medicine? The particulars of the educational program are of less importance to the potential applicant. The faculty is much more knowledgeable than the students in educational matters, and, if they wish to bear the stamp of their influence, they must trust their fate to the faculty's methods and philosophy.

Chapter 5

Medical Education and Practice

M edical schools and their closely affiliated hospitals form medical centers that have as their primary purpose the conversion of untrained manpower into trained manpower.[1] We call this process *education*. Professional education is an expensive process. It requires a large faculty with uncommitted time to interact with the student. The medical center supports a varied and extensive research program, because research is a very effective and, at some stages of development, an essential educational tool. The medical center engages also in giving services to patients because medical practice is also an essential ingredient in the development of a doctor.

The medical center can and does educate a large number of persons. It may even be an efficient producer of manpower. If one views the medical center as a research institute, one immediately highlights inefficiencies in the system. The primary output of a medical center is doctors; the primary output of a research institute is knowledge. The training of doctors to do research results in a higher unit cost for the new knowledge than one needs to pay if they are not teaching students. The medical center may give excellent medical services in terms of the final product. It will not give these excellent services efficiently and at

---

1. Stead EA, Jr. Medical education and practice. *Ann. Int. Med.*, 72:271-274, 1970.

a low unit cost if they are an integral part of the educational program. The use of untrained manpower and the cost in time for converting this green manpower into trained manpower reduces the efficiency of the operation when it is measured in terms of units of service output per dollar. The medical faculty is able to teach in the classroom, to teach in the research laboratory, and to teach in its hospital and clinics because monies have been found to pay the faculty for its total educational effort. There is no magic in the system. Remove the money—stop paying for faculty time, require service to be given efficiently, and require the output of new knowledge to be the major goal of the laboratories in order to balance the budget: the medical center will fail as an educational unit.[2]

In summary, the educational process measured in any terms other than the output of educated doctors will always be expensive and inefficient. The medical schools and their associated medical centers have to live with this fact. They must obtain money to support necessary inefficiencies in research and services when these are used as educational tools. There is nothing to prevent the medical schools and their centers from adding a second component to their operation. They can have some laboratories and some areas of patient service run entirely by trained manpower. A given member of the faculty might want to divide his day: work in the inefficient, education-centered laboratories or clinics for a portion of the day and for the remainder of the day work in the laboratories and clinics using only trained personnel. Some medical centers are toying with this option, but I know none that has fully achieved it.

The community hospital is a place where physicians give ser-

---

2. While this essay was written in 1970, unfortunately, in the year 2000, we are seeing more and more medical centers failing as educational units due to loss of revenue.

vices to people. Money is not available to support a large portion of the staff to interact with students, interns, and residents and to pay for the increase in cost of services, which is unavoidable where service is one of the devices for converting green manpower into trained manpower. The staff of the community hospital is responsible for care in the office, in the home, in the nursing home and extended care units, and in the hospital. The most precious commodity in the doctor's life is time. An internship and residency program in the community hospital saps up the last vestige of time. The doctor attempts to educate the intern and resident, but he soon discovers that he does not have the time to continue his own education. After a tremendous effort, the educational program usually gives little satisfaction to the doctor, to the patient, to the hospital, or to the intern and resident.

During my time as chairman of the departments of medicine at Emory and Duke, I never urged my students to take internships and residencies in community hospitals. The staff of the community hospital is concerned with medicine as it is practiced today. The internship and residency are golden years in which one can learn both the medicine of today and the language and theoretical underpinning of the medicine of tomorrow. No community hospital has the faculty to combine these two elements—the best practice of today and the best preparation for the practice of tomorrow.

There is another strong reason for not supporting extension of the internship and residency programs of the medical center into the community hospital. The problem of the doctor practicing in the community hospital cannot possibly be solved by the intern-resident model. The number of housestaff required to staff this model is greatly in excess of the available total number of interns and residents. In summary, doctors in practice need a clinical support system, but the intern-resident support system does not meet their need.

Five years ago, under my auspices, we decided to experiment with a different type of clinical support system for the practicing physician. We wished to build a stable system that would attract people on a career basis. This person, whom we called a physician's assistant, was to be the "top sergeant" for the doctor. The economics for a support system seemed to be sound if the new member of the team worked in the office, home, and hospital; if the new member worked the same hours as the doctor; and if the new member did tomorrow, on the basis of sound training, many of the things the doctor was doing today. This new member of the doctor's team would extend the arms and eyes of the doctor so that the doctor could accept responsibility for more patients in a given unit of time. For the first time the doctor would have the mechanism—in the person of a stable assistant—for retraining members of his team who were secondary wage earners and who worked intermittently in the health field.

The Duke Department of Medicine structured a 2-year program to train the physician's assistant (PA). In 1967, the program was transferred from the Duke Department of Medicine to the Department of Community and Family Medicine, which was chaired by Dr. E. Harvey Estes. Dr. Robert Howard was the first director of the PA program.

The PA students at Duke are selected by doctors, trained by doctors and, eventually, paid by doctors. The education is related to the medicine of today. The anatomy, physiology, pharmacology, microbiology, and pathology are related to the problems of patients seen in clinical practice. Emphasis is put on the content to be mastered in each different discipline. Biochemistry is not taught as a language that allows the student to read widely and obtain new content whenever he desires it. In the required and elective clinical rotations, emphasis is put on obtaining skills that are to be used in the medicine of today. No attempt is made to prepare the PA for the medicine of tomorrow. This type of apprentice teaching can make any intelligent, interested person capable of carrying out any particular task that the doctor does frequently. When the system is working effectively, the patient cannot know from the performance whether he is being seen by the PA or by the physician. If the PA does the task less skillfully, his training is inadequate and he should not be doing that particular work.

The discovery by the doctor that his assistant can do on any one day the majority of things that he himself does raises some interesting questions about medical education. Why does it take so long to educate the doctor and so little time to educate the assistant?

The doctor's education consists of four parts: (1) preparation to function as a citizen, (2) language preparation so that he can obtain content as needed from books written in part in symbolic languages, (3) development of problem-solving abilities, and (4) application of known knowledge to medical practice.

The society wishes its doctors to have a reasonable knowledge of people, history, social sciences, literature and art because the doctor must relate the mysteries of the human body to the rest of the society. Doctors care for the leaders of our society in times of trouble and, because of the nature of the doctor-patient relationship, doctors can influence the course of the society out of proportion to their actual numbers.

The natural and, hopefully the social, sciences are taught to our doctors because a knowledge of the symbolic languages developed by these disciplines makes a wide variety of content available over the doctor's lifetime. The specific content taught is not important; the ability to read books written in the language of the particular science is important.

The preclinical portion of the doctor's experience serves a

third purpose—namely, to increase problem-solving abilities. Again, the content used to modify the nervous system by having it engage in problem-solving is not important. Practice in problem-solving will modify the nervous system in a favorable way so that problems, regardless of their nature, can be approached more effectively.

The application of known knowledge to the care of people is taught by the apprentice method. This method is very effective for teaching the medicine of today. If one paces the learning correctly and teaches what is not known, one can intersperse apprentice learning with problem solving, use of symbolic language, and acquisition of new content related to the medicine of tomorrow

The overall purpose of the long educational program for doctors is to prepare them for a lifetime of good citizenship and a lifetime of learning. The intent is to create thinking doctors who are completely protected against obsolescence regardless of changes in the social and technological scene.

One can make a first approximation of the success of the educational program by watching the doctor at his daily work. If the doctor has time in the day to be thoughtful, if the doctor can gain new content by the use of training in symbolic language, if the doctor is continually preparing for the medicine of tomorrow, the educational system is justified. If the doctor is harried, tired, handling patients in a routine, non-thinking way, the educational system has failed.

My field survey shows that, in some instances, the doctor in practice meets the expectations of the educational system. The final product has been well worth the time and money invested. In the majority of practices, doctors have been unable to defend their thinking time and their continuing-education time. The practice is carried out in a routinized, non-thinking pattern. The doctor is a harried rather than a thoughtful person. In these instances, the time and money spent on the doctor's education cannot be justified. I had concluded that one had two choices: decrease the time and money spent on the doctor's education, or modify the practice of medicine. One could teach the medical student to perform the medicine of today by the apprentice system and leave out (1) a large part of his general education, (2) the learning of symbolic languages, and (3) problem-solving of a general nature. Obsolescence could be prevented by compulsory apprentice-type retraining each five years. I chose not to take this road because I am still unconvinced that our educational goals are wrong. I believe we use a fine product in the wrong way. Hence my interest in the clinical support systems.

Our PA is structured entirely as a dependent component of the doctor's team. He has no professional existence as an independent agent. A dependent profession is tolerable only if there is a path by which independence is gained. We believe the PA must be dependent to function effectively. His independence must lie in the fact that he can evolve into a doctor. Medical schools will discover that the material covered in the clinical years can be learned before general education, language preparation, and advanced courses in problem-solving are taken. The PA who has worked with patients for a number of years will have clinical knowledge superior to that of the graduating medical student. He should be given credit for this if he wishes to become a doctor.

I am confident that the PA can put time back into the day of the practicing physician, provided the doctor is able to organize his own day and is capable of being a good supervisor[3]. We do not select medical students for their organizing and supervising

---

3. The Physician's Assistant program is now a thriving profession, and every year, National Physician's Assistant day is on October 6, Eugene Stead's Birthday.

talents, and our clinical support system may founder on this hidden reef.

Chapter 6

The Evolution of the Medical University

T he medical school of a generation ago had many of the characteristics of a small college.[1] Its student body was kept relatively homogeneous by rigid admission requirements. The school attempted to transmit to the student a well-defined body of knowledge in both preclinical and clinical areas. It anticipated that most students would have a limited graduate experience and that the school must cover all the facts necessary for the practice of medicine. At graduation, the product was relatively homogeneous, and, in general, each graduate could be replaced by any other graduate. The amount of elective work allowed was small because granting elective time meant leaving out material considered essential by the faculty.

The faculty was small and time to devote to research was limited. The entire effort was directed toward the undergraduate student, and the worth of a faculty member was gauged by his teaching effort. A large investment of faculty time was made to bring along the slower students. The faculty itself was not highly specialized. The reward system emphasized teaching over scholarship.

When a college grows into a university, many changes occur. Students are less homogeneous at entry. They come from wider

1. Stead EA, Jr. The evolution of the medical university. *J. Med. Educ.*, 39:368–373, 1964.

geographical and cultural backgrounds, and they arrive on the campus at widely different stages of training.

The advanced graduate students appear in ever-increasing numbers, and kudos among the faculty are handed out more and more often for research achievements rather than for teaching of undergraduate students. Those students who are slower to mature and who need more individual attention become fewer in number as, gradually, they select smaller, less complex schools.

The faculty of the emerging university becomes increasingly specialized and is willing to accept earlier specialization among the students. The amount of required work is decreased. The faculty, actively engaged in research itself, appreciates the role of research as an educational tool. Students in various honors courses have the opportunity to engage in research as a part of their educational experience. As the number of students spending more than four calendar years in the institution is large, the division between graduate and undergraduate work becomes less rigid. More emphasis is placed on the teaching of mathematics, physics, chemistry, electronics, sociology and psychology as a series of languages, because increasing numbers of students will need to read books written in these symbols.

As these changes in philosophy and practice occur in the educational system, stresses appear in the college social system. The older faculty members feel that there is too much emphasis on research and that too many young staff members teach the introductory undergraduate courses. Moreover, the older members of the college community are sometimes reluctant to give equal status to the increased administrative personnel needed to operate these complex and expensive research ventures. Academic rank becomes less important as the more complex university gives a wider range of rewards.

In the last twenty years, many forces have been at work that have affected the medical scene and produced changes in medical schools. Many of these changes parallel those that occur with the growth of a college into a university.

Doctors drawn together in the military service appreciated the value of group endeavor, both for giving patient care and for continuing education. They returned in large numbers for residency training (graduate medical training) after the war, and, in many medical schools, graduate students for the first time exceeded undergraduate students. The undergraduate student maturing in these schools accepted graduate training as a matter of course, and the average length of medical school contact was gradually lengthened from four years to at least eight years. With the growth of support from the voluntary health agencies and the National Institutes of Health, many full-time faculty positions were established in the clinical departments, and an extensive program of clinical research was begun.

These new faculty members had more uninterrupted time for thinking. They were no longer entirely dependent on patient fees. They could examine in depth the areas of education for which they were responsible. As they worked in the research areas, they could determine the adequacy of their training for research. They realized that relatively little research is done as a doctor. The M.D. training gives one access to patients and an appreciation of the number of unknown variables that go into patient care. When the physician attempts to add new facts to the body of medical knowledge, however, he must function as a scientist and use the language and methodology of one or more of the scientific disciplines. Doctors responsible for large research programs began to urge their graduate students to spend less time in standard clinical training and more time in mastering the language of mathematics, chemistry, physics, electronics, psychology, sociology and communications. They wanted the trainees responsible for clinical research in the future to have had a rich research experience involving some area of quantitative biology. This could be accomplished only by a marked expansion in the basic science departments in the medical school and by more cooperation between the science departments of the medical school and the other science areas of the university.

An appreciation of the importance of basic science training and of the importance of physicists, engineers, biochemists, geneticists, mathematicians, psychologists, and other scientists in solving problems of biology was hastened by the development of the intramural program of the National Institutes of Health. Many of the brightest young trainees with M.D. degrees spent their two years of service time in this intramural program. For this two-year period, the customary rapid post-graduation movement to ever-increasing clinical responsibility was broken. Many of these young physicians had a type of experience that they would never have selected voluntarily, because it was outside the cultural pattern of the usual M.D. program. But, being bright and accustomed to hard work, they rapidly adapted to their new role as scientists. When they returned to the medical schools — many as faculty members — they brought with them a different notion of the role of the non-medical scientist in the medical world. Coming up against career researchers, they had gained an appreciation for the need of a good knowledge of scientific language as a prerequisite for a career in which they expected support from the research dollar.

With the increased emphasis on research, funds were available for enlarging the basic science departments. Because of the needs of the whole health field, faculty could be supported beyond the needs of the school to impart information to undergraduate medical students. With the increased sophistication of the clinicians in many areas of basic science, and with the recognition of the importance of the basic sciences as training bases for the future, medical schools began to appoint students of distinction to their basic science departments who were more interested in general biology than in the immediate problems of disease. Clinicians interested in research supported the appointment of able scientists with non-clinical interests, because these clinicians understood that the laboratories of such scientists would be ideal for the training of physician-scientists. The basic science faculty members had been closely allied to their university graduate schools before being recruited into medical schools. They began, therefore, within the framework of the medical school, to develop Ph.D. programs in their own areas of special interest. In many instances, faculty of the basic science departments spend more man-hours of instruction on their predoctoral fellows than on their medical students.

While these changes in the faculty were evolving, the student body was also changing. Premedical advisers and students were beginning to identify medical schools as an appropriate place for training in quantitative biology. For the first time, the schools began to have students with advanced training in mathematics, chemistry, physics, psychology, sociology, engineering and electronics who intended to use this training for the study of biological processes. These students with a good command of the scientific language were intermixed with students with majors in English, history, philosophy, economics and languages. who had a limited ability to read books written in scientific symbols. The medical school did not want to narrow their intake. Their role was to supply manpower for the whole health field. The non-scientist who wishes to give service to his fellow-man will treat many more sick persons than the quantitative biologist who is interested in how man functions in health and disease. Conversely, the scientist will serve few patients with his own hands, but he will create new knowledge which will increase greatly the effectiveness of the practicing doctor.

Much of the pressure for changing our ways has come from clinical specialists. They wish to train two types of specialists:

those who apply what is known and those who make major contributions of new knowledge to the specialty. At the level of applied knowledge, all clinical specialties are narrow; at the level of scientific disciplines useful in solving the unknown problems, all specialties are as broad as science. The clinical specialist interested in training doctors with a broad base in the scientific disciplines underlying the specialty, found that the time the candidate could invest in training was exhausted before he reached the specialty area.

The increasing heterogeneity of the student body and the differing goals of the students has posed unanswerable problems for the medical college. Calculus could not be used in the teaching of physiology or chemistry, because many of the students did not understand that language. Biochemistry could not be taught as an advanced course, because many of the students had not had a thorough grounding in chemistry. Many students with a strong desire to be a doctor had little interest in science as such, and were puzzled by the insistence that they learn material that, clearly, practicing doctors did not use. The solution in most schools has been to use the four medical school years for a general survey of the medical field. This solution allows all of the medical students to have a common experience regardless of their preparation, but it produces no student who has really mastered any one discipline. The internship is one more year of general experience. Then come two years in the service and one more year of refresher work before young doctors decide to specialize in a clinical area. They still have time to learn what the current specialist does in clinical practice, but they have spent too much time in general areas to master one or more of the scientific disciplines that allows them to make major contributions in their field of special interest. Their trouble cannot be that they have not put in enough years. They have spent four years in college surveying; four years in medical school surveying; and four years in hospitals and the service surveying. Unfortunately, by the time the surveying is over, they may be too old to learn.

As the small homogeneous medical college faculty differentiates into the heterogeneous faculty of specialists of various sorts, and as new careers open for people in the health field, some medical schools will evolve into medical universities. They will accept their role as producers of a wide variety of doctors, both M.D.'s and Ph.D.'s, to meet the needs of the health field. They will adapt their curricula to maintain the heterogeneity of their intake and will not be perturbed by the fact that their output, too, is heterogeneous. They will allow early specialization and will no longer insist that each medical student have the same experiences in medical school as every other student. A curriculum will develop along the following lines: All the material in the basic sciences essential to the practice of medicine will be given in the first year of medical school. This material will be presented in terms that can be understood by the student body possessing diverse language preparations. In the second year, students will be placed on the wards of a general hospital to find out what doctors actually do; they will determine at this point whether they want to devote themselves primarily to patient care, using the information medicine now has, or whether they want to acquire a scientific background that will allow them to create new knowledge.[2]

At the end of their second year, students will have satisfied all the terms of the bond. They are now free to differentiate in any way they like. If they wish to follow a scientific path and are deficient in the language of mathematics or biochemistry, students can use the resources of the university to master the language deficiency. If they wish to use their skill as engineers to

---

2. These changes are in essence those that were implemented in the Duke medical school curriculum in the early 1960s.

work on problems related to servomechanisms, they may take little or no more clinical work. If they wish to be physicians and have demonstrated little interest in science divorced from clinical care, they will learn best from patient problems and will have the remainder of their basic science experiences centered around problems originating in patients.

In essence, students after the second year will work with their committees that are responsible for helping them with career planning. This committee will be free to use the entire resources of the university, including the medical center, to reach the desired goal. Students will be working toward their own goals and will put more energy into the project than if they were working toward an impersonal general curriculum. It will now be possible to plan in depth a period of at least six years. This includes the last two years of medical school, two years of graduate training, and two years of service time. By proper planning, the service time can be used for laboratory training or for clinical training. The services have many places that are best filled by persons who have made a career choice and have begun the process of differentiation.

With the tremendous growth in the health field and with the increasing specialization in both biological sciences and clinical areas, pressure has mounted to create new departments in the medical school. In the past, each new department required fixed space in the curriculum and, unless the number of departments was limited, the student's time was hopelessly fragmented. With a core curriculum limited to two years, and with the rest of the time elective, the curriculum need no longer act as a brake on the creation of new departments.

At one end of the medical school, the basic science faculty will be firmly anchored with the graduate school of the university and with the departments of the undergraduate schools that supply advanced students for the basic science departments. It will handle the basic science core courses for the medical students and serve as a training base for scientists at all levels in the medical center. At the other end will be the clinicians taking care of patients and teaching students at all levels how to give this care. Slowly, a new segment of the faculty is growing up: a group of physician-scientists who are primarily supported by the research dollar because of the special needs of the health field. These faculty see patients in selected areas and carry the problems of these patients back to the laboratory. This portion of the faculty is becoming increasingly responsible for teaching the students at all levels those portions of the various scientific disciplines that are easily learned from observations on patients. Such faculty hold joint appointments in clinical and preclinical departments.

The growth of the medical school from a fixed curriculum, centered about the production of a standard product, into a more flexible program, centered around graduate education, will develop most profitably where the medical school is an integral part of the university campus. The medical school will need university help with its graduate students, particularly in the areas of mathematics, biology, psychology, sociology, physics, engineering and chemistry. The numerous and sophisticated faculty accumulated in the health area will give many courses that will attract not only predoctoral fellows and medical students but various groups of honor students at the undergraduate level. The medical school will still exist as an identifiable area producing doctors, but its students will work throughout the university, and students from other parts of the university will use the facilities of the medical center. This program will emphasize the unity of scholarly attitude that is at the heart of a medical university, rather than the unity of current information characteristic of the medical college.

Finally, to the university presidents: The health professions are certain to become the largest users of trained manpower in the world. Because of the demands of the people, money will continue to come into this area more easily than into many other fields. Universities and medical schools have not wished to face the tremendous demand for trained manpower in the health field, nor have they realized their inability to meet this tide with their present facilities. Properly used, this surge offers a great challenge for university development. The day will pass when university presidents are pitied for the headaches posed by their health area. Instead, they will be envied for the opportunities for general university development opened up by their medical centers.

Chapter 7

The Limitations of Teaching

I n our most productive clinical graduate programs, the interns and residents have been teachers of undergraduate students and of themselves.[1] The profit accruing from this combined teaching-learning process is evident by the degree of excellence achieved by the doctors produced by these programs. In recent years, the suggestion has been made that permanent faculty members be paid for recycling each quarter the introductory material that has proven such an excellent base for consolidation of the thoughts and ideas of the junior revolving staff. This means appointing clinical faculty primarily as teachers. This matter is of sufficient importance at the present time to warrant detailed consideration.

What are the teaching needs of a clinical service? Clinical departments need teachers to help in transferring to their students information present in books. They need, also, teachers who are going to present to the student a clear picture of what is not known about biological systems and who can inspire and lead the student to prepare himself to solve some of these puzzling and interesting problems.

On any clinical service, one finds a number of bright young residents who are very effective teachers of the current state of the art. They are capable doctors, completely trustworthy and

---

1. Stead EA, Jr. The limitations of teaching. *Pharos*, 32:54-57, 1969.

loved by both patients and students. They are interested in what is known. They have nothing they want to contribute to extend existing knowledge, and they have no stimulus to use scientific journals to communicate with their colleagues. As they teach their colleagues, they learn that each person has a personalized receiving system and an individualized processing system. They make the discovery that they can never predict the effect of any input into the nervous system of another man by any form of theoretical calculation. They have to listen to the playback from the system receiving the input to determine the degree of change produced. This information is of incalculable value in the practice of medicine.

When we allow these currently effective teachers to move into practice without a marked effort to hold them in the university, we are severely criticized by our students at both the undergraduate and graduate level. We are accused of killing off teachers by the "publish or perish" attitude. We are told that we should reward good teaching by academic tenure, early promotion and good pay. I have never believed that it is desirable to add persons to the permanent faculty because they are good and effective teachers. Since this point of view is now strongly criticized by others, I will give my reasons for holding to this staid and supposedly outdated position.

When we add a new faculty member, we are potentially making a lifelong commitment. If we select them primarily for their teaching ability, we have decided to use them as teachers for the duration of their lives. We have selected them not for their other attributes but for their teaching abilities. The problem inherent in this basis of selection is in the fact that few teachers remain maximally effective as teachers over their full professional lifetime. Moreover, there is no way to determine that any teacher actually achieves what is arbitrarily defined as good teaching. In the medical center we are dealing with a group of bright medical students interested in successful professional careers. They will learn a great deal no matter what the teachers do. Certainly we would be foolish to pay a teacher for what is going to happen without him.

The effectiveness of the teacher must be judged by the things that happen after the student and teacher part company. The immediate communication between student and teacher is usually of more benefit to the teacher than to the student.

The interchange causes teachers to order their thoughts. The movement and rearrangement of material stored in their memory increases the chance for the stored knowledge to be transformed into usable, easily available knowledge and may even evoke an original thought. Usually the student forgets the material unless the contact causes him to undertake intellectual work he would not have done without the student-teacher interaction. This brings us to the hard fact that effective teaching is an interaction and can be prevented by the student, the teacher or both. A casual glance at this frame of reference will convince us that any one teacher cannot be an effective teacher to all students.

All students are differential receivers with personalized processing systems. In terms of enzymology, the teacher must change the student substrate into its activated form. Most of the energy required for reaching the activated state must come from the student. Since students are undergoing continual change, all teachers who cannot continue to undergo equal change will gradually become less effective. In practice, few teachers can survive competition from their bright youngsters for longer than ten years. Shall we employ a faculty to be effective teachers for ten years and dull old men and women for the next 30 years? How can one identify the long-lived teachers and thus avoid the boredom present in many schools?

The teacher more interested in conveying attitudes will survive longer than the teacher interested in transmitting facts.

Teaching young doctors how to acknowledge their mistakes and how to learn from them without wasting energy defending their errors is a good example. Learning how to learn easily from an error has more general applicability than the transmission of any known fact.

The teacher more concerned with what is not known about a subject will have a longer survival than one who makes the transmission of current knowledge his primary goal. The student is more likely to make moves on his own if he is exploring carefully the validity of the premises on which current practice is based than if he is learning what is the best current practice.

The teacher at the bedside who gives a discourse on what he knows about the matter will come off second best to the teacher who identifies the problem presented by the patient and arranges material relevant to the problem in three phases: (a) what the student and other persons present know about the identified problem and what the teacher can add; (b) what is certainly available in the library and can be learned by having each member of the group collect some of the appropriate information; and (c) what is likely not to be yet known about the problem but could now be learned because of developments in science that have occurred since the problem was last intensively studied.

The teacher who listens well will survive longer than the one who parrots the same record each time the button is pushed.

The teacher who, as a matter of pride in his own ability, listens carefully to define areas for intellectual exploration when the resident says this patient is of little interest, will have a longer survival.

Teachers who get up in the morning determined to learn something about biological or biosocial systems that they did not know yesterday will have to undergo continual change and, therefore, increase their chances of staying in touch with their students. It makes no difference how this drive expresses itself. It may be in the clinic or the laboratory. In years gone by, when there were few financial rewards for research, this quality was present in most people engaged in laboratory work. Therefore, a departmental chairman selecting a faculty member for a long teaching life chose one with research experience. Now that there are financial rewards for laboratory work, one has to be much more cautious in use of this criterion.

Teachers who do not take themselves too seriously and who are willing to be replaced by able youngsters when they pass them in any area will live a longer life as teachers than the ones who are destroyed by the fact that eventually they must become less important to the institution.

Effective teachers must be able to make demands on others. They cannot be paralyzed by their own inadequacies and failures. They must require excellence from their students at all times. Effort and good intentions are not enough. The students must be judged by their achievement and the students must learn the difference between success and failure.

Effective teachers are happy teachers. They count their blessings even though they know life is not perfect. They appreciate the frailties of man and his organizations but spend little of their energies bemoaning them. They will die for only certain things. Most of the time they will walk around obstructions and not bloody their noses unnecessarily.

The most effective and long-lived teachers create an atmosphere in which intellectual achievement has honor. The teacher shares with his student the fun and satisfaction created by the intellectual achievement of the student. The returns to the student for his effort create enough pleasurable feelings for him to want to repeat the process. This is the way to develop a pattern of lifetime learning. The creation of the environment where learning has honor and produces satisfaction is a more important function of the faculty than the creation of libraries, laboratories or classrooms.

The most long-lived teachers are those who best understand the limitations of teaching. When teachers work, they gain knowledge. When students work, they gain knowledge. The crossover is very small. Teachers are useful because they create the physical and intellectual setting where the student works and because they can tell the student whether or not his performance has achieved excellence. They can lead the student to look into areas he does not know about. They can identify books that are useful to read. They can point out that the student has examined only one side of a problem. They can lead the student to realize that he has accepted unproven assumption as proven facts. They can determine whether the student has prepared himself to read the books that will be useful to him. Teachers are most useful when the student is active. The more active the teacher, the less the learning opportunity for the student.

The most effective teachers create a shadowy framework in which the student can climb. If teachers fill in the skeleton in great detail, they will limit the learning by their own knowledge. If they make the form recognizable but leave the final shape and details to the student, the student may produce a much better intellectual synthesis than the teacher. A teacher may be likened to an artist. A pedestrian artist may produce an exact copy of a scene and most viewers will see approximately the same thing. The picture will not live because it will have little relevance to the changing patterns of life. A much less precise picture, suggesting a mother and child while leaving many details to the imagination, will come to life in as many interpretations as there are viewers. Some of these interpretations may be superior to the original concept of the artist. This impressionist quality of a teacher can be assayed. Skilled teachers never have any difficulty in teaching students together who are at widely different stages in the learning process. They give some new facts to the beginners; they lead the intermediate group to incorporate the facts in a new framework; and they stimulate the advanced students to relate the new frame of reference to phenomena that they have puzzled about in the past. They leave behind them an agreed-upon allocation of tasks where each person will have to try his hand at ordering and transmitting information because they will have the responsibility for teaching someone else.

The most long-lived and effective teachers can tolerate ignorance. When students are thoughtfully exploring an area new to them, they cannot be penalized if they are ignorant of yet unexplored areas. People who must know every fact, who are destroyed if they must admit ignorance, are at the mercy of everyone who asks them a question. Too much memory work makes original thinking impossible. Memory is the accumulation of facts; thinking is the manipulation of facts. Many facts are best left in books. The best clinician conducts thinking ward rounds, not memory ward rounds. The goal of teaching is to create independence. To achieve this aim, long-lived teachers assume two roles. In the administrative role, they are the leaders and maintain the discipline that permits the learning situation to develop. In the learning situation there is no administrative hierarchy. The leader is the one who can best manipulate the relevant facts and procedures to solve the problem. Students will cautiously test the teachers to see if they can tolerate intellectual freedom. If they can, the goal of education may be met.

Teachers who survive a long time know their limitations and are careful not to be destructive. They know that young people mature and grow. These young people will accomplish many things without teachers. They often give the teacher the credit because they are not experts in the learning process and a teacher they like happens to be standing by. The non-participating role of the teacher is shown clearly if, years later, student and teacher discuss the matter. The student can remember clearly every detail of the great moment when a new period of personal or intellectual growth started. The teacher is completely blank. Certainly he had no inkling at the time that a major event was occurring and he had no way to fix the event in his mind. I know of no thoughtful teacher or leader of the young who has not been embarrassed by the credit given him for words and acts which have completely passed from his memory. The teacher can take one thing to his credit: he did not stop the development. I have said enough about the complexity of the problem, and I have stated my belief that selecting faculty for teaching ability will only make your institution dull. Well—then what?

Teaching should be the price of admission to the club and not something to be paid for over the period in which you belong to the faculty. If one is neither a good teacher nor wishes to become one, he should not be given a place on the faculty of a medical school. The school should appoint faculty for their excellence in research, their skill in patient care, their ability to write and communicate, their capacity for leadership and administration. Everyone should do some teaching, and this should be for love and not for pay. There shouldn't be adequate money in the budget to pay a portion of the faculty each year for giving more time to teaching than is required for admission to the club. Assignment to the teaching budget should be on a yearly basis, and each faculty member should know that the time will come when he will be replaced by younger faculty. The teaching budget should pay for time over and beyond that contributed by the average faculty member, but each faculty so supported should know that, over his lifetime, he cannot expect major support from the teaching budget. Departments who add staff solely because of their teaching ability, expecting to support them as teachers over their active life, create very dull shops. An occasional faculty member will break the mold. When that happens, enjoy them but do not build your house on this unlikely-to-be-found rock. The best intern and residency programs will incorporate the interns and residents in the teaching program. The faculty will watch these young housestaff teach and will reward them appropriately for teaching during their years as junior faculty members.

Chapter 8

Training Is No Substitute for Education

The current interest in North Carolina to prepare its young people for the work force by vocational schooling makes a review of the differences between education and training timely.[1] The words *education* and *training* are frequently used interchangeably. We need to appreciate the differences and similarities between these two modalities and not confuse one with the other.

In a narrow sense, education and training have the same goals. Each attempts to establish in the central nervous system new learning patterns which facilitate the performance of new tasks and improve the performance of previously-learned tasks. An educational program attempts to produce a wide range of changes in the nervous system and to increase the general capacity of the neural network to store information and to move and rearrange facts. We use the word *memory* to describe the acquisition and storage of information and the word *thinking* to describe the movement and rearrangement of countless bits of information.

The goal of education is to enlarge and extend the many functional neural networks of the brain for greater storage and processing of information. Such networks cover a wide range of content: language, culture, history, art, music, science, feeling

1. Stead EA, Jr. Training is no substitute for education. *North Carolina Medical Journal*, 45:579-580, 1984.

states, religion, mathematics, communication, etc. A fully educated brain contains innumerable hooks for attaching, rearranging, and using the information accumulated in the memory system. It can identify problems and solve them. The brain is attuned to profit by history, by knowledge of the great religions, and by the roles that feeling states and culture play in the affairs of man. Education strives to develop a brain capable of enjoying the day and to improve the capacity of the brain to tolerate without hostility the belief systems and behavior of other persons. Education can make the day more enjoyable; the outcome of education is useful when it creates attitudes and feelings that make the day more meaningful.

The educational process is not necessarily related to the production of useful things. Training develops the neural pathways formed by education into well-grooved and well-worn tracks that permit repetitive performances with a high degree of efficiency. Training is aimed at the formation of habits that are so ingrained by repetition that only a minimal outlay of nervous energy is required for performance. Training leads to efficiency over a narrow spectrum; education leads to a broader spectrum of competency.

High school, college, the early years of medical school, and experiences in research laboratories are oriented toward education. Internships and residencies are designed to train the doctor to perform repetitious tasks efficiently. Many postgraduate posts combine research (education) with clinical activities (training).

Our high schools tend to be divided into those that prepare students for college and those that prepare students for direct entry into the work force. The latter are called vocational schools. Graduates from either type of high school will move to areas where it is hoped they will continue to learn. Graduates from high school entering the work force will be trained on the job to perform tasks required by their work. In most instances there will be little time for unstructured educational programs. Their continued education depends on individual effort in an unstructured environment. The only educational capital they have is that obtained during their high school years. They pay a penalty if their vocational high school has sacrificed education for training.

High school graduates going to college have a better chance of continuing their education, depending on whether the faculty of the college they have selected comprehends the difference between the words *education* and *training*. Eventually college graduates enter the work force. If their brain has been altered in a favorable way by their college experiences, they will be quicker to see opportunities beyond their first job. Their college education should protect them to some extent from the rapid changes of our modern society and technology.

At high school graduation we hope that students have the following attributes:

1. A picture of themselves as those who are capable of earning a living in our society.
2. An ability to enjoy the day and not resent the fact that others can legitimately make demands on them.
3. The ability to work with concentration at a task until it is complete.
4. An awareness of time in terms of punctuality and as a measure of efficiency.
5. An appreciation of the fact that the teacher as well as the student has problems.
6. The ability to read English with speed and comprehension. They should be able to understand written instructions quickly and correctly.
7. The ability to communicate accurately by written and spoken word.

8. A quantitative sense which allows them to use mathematics to solve problems and to make accurate measurements.
9. An overview of the arts and sciences which allows them to comprehend books in these areas written for the general public.
10. An adequate knowledge of history which lets them know the complexity of our social, political and economic systems.
11. An ethical sense that distinguishes between right and wrong and supplies a framework for continued personal growth.

High school graduates with this educational background can enter the work force of modern society free from fears of obsolescence. Education, not training, protects their futures.

Vocational education was formalized because a number of students did not appreciate the need for an educational program and wished task-oriented training which would equip them to earn immediate income. We have always had this problem in medical schools. Some students want to learn only those aspects of biomedical science that are most quickly applied to clinical problems. In the clinical years they wish to be trained for clinical tasks rather than to explore new areas of knowledge which will be applicable clinically in later years. The wise instructor uses the least amount of task-oriented material that is compatible with holding the attention of the student. He leads the student to explore knowledge tangential to the current task, which prepares the student for the future. The faculty know that in most instances the total intellectual capital of the student will be accumulated before he enters private practice. Training continues in practice but education frequently stops. A recent publication of the National Academy of Sciences[2] entitled *High Schools and the Changing Workplace* addresses the differences between education and training. It emphasizes the weakness of the predominantly vocational approach and urges that today's high schools guard against selling the student's educational birthright for a mess of vocational porridge.

2. *High Schools and the Changing Workplace. The Employee's View.* Report of the Panel on Secondary School Education for the Changing Workplace. National Academy Press, Washington, DC, 1984.

Chapter 9

Making Safe Doctors

The Duke Medical School has been unusually successful because a reasonable portion of the faculty has avoided the temptation of cramming into four years all of the material that the doctor will find useful during a lifetime of practice.[1] Other schools insist on four years of memorization under the guise that this is necessary to produce "safe doctors."

We know that any doctor who knows what he or she knows and can comfortable say, "I don't know," is a safe doctor. Duke has thus been able to comfortably give its students degrees of freedom not available in other schools. The school has the opportunity to use the undergraduate years to expand the language capabilities of its students and to pass them on to a large variety of careers with an improved neural network.

The basic science faculty are in the fortunate position of not being bound by content. They can extend the joy of learning and involve the students in a large variety of experiences. They can teach them to read the languages of the molecular biologist the immunologist, the biochemist, the anatomist, the bacteriologist, the physiologist, and the pathologist and open the door to life-long learning. Since the majority of the students will not become professionals in these disciplines, the faculty can avoid

---

1. Stead EA, Jr. Making safe doctors, unpublished essay. Presented at the Duke Medical Alumni Association, 1983.

the drills necessary to establish habits that allow one to perform in an area without thinking.

The clinical faculty is less free. They must begin the formation of habit patterns that will be used every day in practice. They do not have to complete this process to the exclusion of all else. They still have the opportunity to improve the neural network and to allow the student to learn at his own pace, always protected by the ability to say, "I don't know but if it's important I will learn it." Because Duke has been willing to limit the number of facts to be memorized in medical school, its students and residents are able to use research as one of its educational tools. Medical students can spend a full year in research and graduate with their class. Residents combining research and clinical training are given special consideration, and in many areas, full credit for the research years. Duke has recognized the impact of debt on the freedom of young physicians and allows medical students to receive both pay and scholastic credit for a year in the laboratory.

Freedom has been a rewarding experience to many Duke students—but freedom is difficult to maintain. There has always been a portion of the Duke faculty who believe that the content of the basic sciences must be drilled into medical students and that the function of the basic science years is to change the brain into a memorized text book. The demonstration that the other schools pursuing this course have not been successful does not deter them. They want to go back to two years of lectures—unmindful of the forgetting curve.

Chapter 10

The Role of Science and of the Belief Systems of Patients and Doctors in the Practice of Medicine

O nly a portion of the medical care in this country is given by persons trained in the scientific method. The fact that a large number of persons believe they benefit from a wide variety of non-scientific healers must mean that there are ways of helping people that to date have defied scientific analysis.[1] In actuality, the gulf between scientific healers and non-scientific healers is smaller than is usually appreciated. Scientifically-trained healers hope to treat completely understood illnesses by the use of science. But there are few completely understood diseases and even those we understand occur in persons whose bodies differ dramatically from patient-to-patient because of genetic and environmental effects. The practice of the most rigid scientific doctor is composed of a mixture or what is called the art and science of medicine. The art is the sum of activities that result from the interaction of the brains of the doctor and the patient. Each year a small modicum of practice moves from the poorly understood area of the art into the area of scientific practice.

---

1. Stead EA, Jr. The role of science and of the belief systems of patient and doctors in the practice of medicine, unpublished essay. October 15, 1980.

Most non-M.D. healers engage only in the art and do not have the scientific backup. Most doctors with the scientific back-up actually use more art than science. There is no simple way of knowing what will happen in the central nervous system. Until late in an illness that is destroying an organ, incapacity is more likely to occur from the perception of the person with the disease than from the disease itself. Improvement may occur because of improvement in the organ or from changes in the way the brain evaluates the total situation.

The scientific healer knows that improvement or worsening of the patient can come from changes in peripheral organs or from changes in perception. The non-scientific healer rarely knows enough about the nervous system to appreciate that improved overall function may occur with no change in the diseased organ. He believes that his art has changed the amount of disease and does not know that the likely answer is that his art has had its primary effect on the brain.

Scientifically-trained doctors have usually not wished to study human behavior. Few doctors know much about sex and even fewer have studied the effects of drugs outside the laboratory. Our notions of right and wrong are seriously at risk when we study behavior that may erode our notions of right and wrong. Avoidance is the safest course. Examination of non-scientific healing has been on this same restricted basis. The scientific doctor in his reductionist manner examines the healing process in a narrow framework of reference. If he discovers that the chiropractic does not really produce dramatic changes in the structure of the spine, he is satisfied to say that the chiropractic is a quack. The fact that the patient functions better and is pleased to pay this non-scientific healer is overlooked. A more curious frame of reference and a willingness to accept the fact that improvement may come from a variety of causes might lead to more interesting results.

I was amazed at the way the laetril controversy[2] was handled. The scientific physician rapidly guessed that this material would not hurt cancer cells and dismissed the whole affair out of hand. It is very likely that an interested team of observers caring for 200 patients who elected this treatment would have learned a great deal about human behavior and the brain.

Persons interested in music, dance, and exercise programs believe that they can change the state of the body and improve health in many people. Does improvement come from changes in bones, nerves and muscles, or does it come from chemicals produced peripherally or centrally which change the brain and improve the patient's view of self.

The time has come to develop a few areas in this country where ideas about health and illness from a variety of cultures can be observed. Those that are beneficial can be used at once even if the cause of the benefit is still not identified. Those that have no benefit can be identified. There are now available ways to identify and compare certain changes and to compare results from different approaches. Biofeedback and dance can be compared for their ability to produce relaxation in a variety of muscles. The serenity noted in our exercising enthusiasts can be compared with that created by a visit to an art museum or concert. The effect of meditation on electroencephalographic patterns during the day and night can be compared with those produced by exercise. The production of hormones by the brain under different modalities of treatment can be followed.

Would any scientifically-oriented medical center be willing to study what can be learned from the examination of this great

---

2. Laetril was an alternative medicine cancer treatment made from apricot pits that was dismissed by mainstream medicine. It was subsequently proven to not be effective for cancer treatment, but not before many patients took the treatment.

variety of belief systems? This is a venture for the private rather than the public sector. Will any foundation or group of foundations support this venture? I suggest that the time has come for a small conference to examine these questions.[3]

---

3. This essay is from 1980 and now 20 years later, the Duke Integrative Medicine Center has been founded to systemically study the effectiveness of a variety of "alternative medicine" treatments.

Chapter 11

A Curious, Interested Doctor at Peace with the Complexities of Biology

I enjoyed reading Drew's account[1] of the principles of drug monitoring.[2] Molecular change at the site of action of a drug is the final culmination of a series of distribution curves, each with a wide base. I remember the excitement when the purified glycosides of digitalis leaf became available. One distribution curve, namely the amount of active agent in each pill, was narrowed. Because of the differences in preparation of the pills, the amount of drug available for absorption varied widely. The distribution curves of bioavailability have a broad base and purification of the glycoside was of little help until the base of this curve was narrowed by better formulation by the pharmaceutical industry.

We then ran into a new set of distribution curves. The rate of disappearance from the blood and the degree of attachment of the active drug to cell membranes and cellular structures showed wide variability. The desired hemodynamic effects were not readily predicted by the serum levels. Drew states some of the

---

1. Drew RH. A new era in pharmacotherapy: The need to understand the principles of therapeutic drug monitoring. *North Carolina Medical Journal*, 45:213-217, 1984.

2. Stead EA, Jr. A curious, interested doctor at peace with the complexities of biology. *North Carolina Medical Journal*, 45:251, 1984.

reasons for this. Digitalis levels do allow us to identify our non-compliant patients and the patients who have a level that produces toxicity in the majority of patients. This is, of course, progress.

We know that a series of distribution curves determine the way the kidney excretes the drug. We know that the free level of the drug is altered by many other drugs. There must be at least 50 more distribution curves to be mastered before we can accurately define in quantitative terms the effects of digitalis.

Students of all types come to us to learn the science of clinical medicine. To me scientific medicine is a situation in which the doctor can control all the variables, elect a course and, after an absence of a number of days, return to find that the patient has stayed on the course charted by the doctor. Because of the complexity of biology with its thousands of overlapping distribution curves, this is rarely possible. I would rather have a doctor who continually observes the patient's course, knowing the depths of his ignorance, than a doctor who looks on himself as a scientist capable of controlling all the variables. An alert, curious, interested doctor who is at peace with the complexity of biology is a great asset to patients.

Kenneth Melman, a distinguished clinical pharmacologist, makes the same point in a paper entitled "Will the Sighted Physician See?"[3] If we behave inappropriately we will continually press for miracle agents that do only good. Yet, in demanding substantial efficacy we are *asking* for chemical agents that intervene substantially in biological processes. Such agents used thoughtlessly or wrongly will produce disease. If we fail to think through this problem we will miss out on one of the biggest and most exciting challenges of medicine. That challenge is to

---

3. Melman, KL. Will the sighted physician see? *The Pharos*, 47:2-6, 1984.

observe the unexpected, to analyze it in the light of our knowledge and determine if we are truly seeing something new. It is the physician's privilege to observe biology in man, a model never fully replicated by laboratory animals.

II

Academic Medical Centers

My own belief is that the genetic approach offers the opportunity for the preventive medicine of the future. Genetic backgrounds will determine the disease states that can be activated by the environment. Preventive medicine will modify the environment for the particular person to prevent the development of the unfavorable genetic possibilities.

Chapter 12

Retooling Clinical Departments in Academic Health Centers

I t has been my good fortune to have had sixteen years as chairman of a department of medicine — first at Emory University and, for the last twelve years, at Duke.[1] During this time we have had a significant influence on medical education, not only at Emory and Duke but over a broader area as well. From our services, Paul Beeson[2] has gone to Yale, Jack Myers[3] to Pittsburgh, Sam Martin[4] to Gainesville, John Hickam[5] to Indiana,

---

1. Stead EA, Jr. A request for funds for the retooling and orderly expansion of the Department of Medicine at Duke University. A proposal for Dr. Barnes Woodhall, Vice President and Dean, Duke Medical Center, 1959.

2. Paul Beeson, M.D. was with Dr. Stead at Emory (1942-1947), and was Physician-in-Chief and Chair, Department of Medicine at Yale School of Medicine from 1952-1965.

3. Jack Myers, M.D. was in Dr. Stead's department at Emory (1942-1947) and at Duke (1947-1955), and was Chief of Medicine at the University of Pittsburgh from 1955-1970.

4. Sam Martin, M.D. was the first Chief Resident appointed at Duke by Dr. Stead. He later became Professor of Medicine and Dean at the University of Florida, Gainesville.

5. John Hickam, M.D. was Chair and Professor of Medicine at the University of Indiana Medical School.

and James Warren[6] to Galveston. All these men, now chairman of their respective departments, have built or are building units like the one at Duke which I have described. All of them have taken Duke and Emory trainees along with them, so that our philosophy of learning has become widespread.

As the activities of the last sixteen years are reviewed, a central theme becomes obvious. At Emory our first assignment was to arrange the department's teaching program within the blocks of time allotted to the Department of Medicine. We decided first to free the faculty of any compulsion to cover a very large block of knowledge. We would teach from the patients and attach knowledge already acquired to the particular patient the student was caring for. The student would reinvestigate those phases of the basic sciences that applied to the particular patient and learn that part of clinical medicine that applied to the same patient. The patient would be the stimulus for learning, because this stimulus would last as long as the student practiced medicine. The role of the faculty would be to see that the student enjoyed his learning experiences and developed a desire to continue them. This system of "slow" learning required that the faculty be willing to tolerate ignorance of many specific areas of medicine. If we laid down no hard and fast body of knowledge that had to be learned, we could not criticize students for ignorance of a particular fact. We had to base our judgments on their ability to use those facts they did have. If they could manipulate these facts, tear them down and rebuild new structures with them — in short, think — we would be satisfied.

---

6. James Warren, M.D. was a long-time colleague and collaborator of Gene Stead's, who co-authored the classic Stead paper explaining the pathophysiology of congestive heart failure in *Archives of Internal Medicine,* 73:138-147, 1944.

My Emory students are now well-established in practice, teaching and research. I have heard from them often about their experiences as interns at other hospitals. They realized that they had memorized fewer facts than students from many other schools; but they were not dismayed when new situations arose and they were satisfied with their ability to learn from each new experience. I am satisfied that their performance since graduation indicates the method by which they were taught was successful.

Thus, my Emory years were spent in freeing the members of the department from the need for compulsive coverage of the field of internal medicine and in freeing medical students from the idea that they worked because they were in school. Instead, students learned to work for the fun of learning and to give their patients good care.

During my Duke experience I have had time to extend my educational interests. We have worked hard at the intern level. The intern year, we felt, should accomplish two things. First, it should give the intern a hard core of carefully thought-out and worked over knowledge, which would serve as a crystal to which additional knowledge could be attached. Second, the intern must be freed from the compulsion to develop all phases of a patient's work-up with equal care.

To achieve the first goal—a hard core of knowledge—interns are exposed to two types of experience; they participate in student teaching where they must defend their own ideas to their peers, and they present their ideas on the behavior of their patients and pathogenesis of disease processes to senior members of the staff.

In pursuit of our second aim—to train interns to use reason in the work-up of their patients—we are aided by necessity. In the fourth year, students carry a small patient load and have time for synthesis and correlation. At that level they can spend equal time on all phases of the history and examination. As interns, they must develop quick clinical reflexes and carry a heavy workload. They must now learn to distribute their time unevenly. It is no longer possible to put equal time on each part of the history and examination. This experience breaks down the training routines learned in the third and fourth years. Interns find they can handle simple problems rapidly and simply, and so have the time they need for complicated problems.

During my years at Emory, I was impressed by the fact that our best Grady Hospital (the city hospital of Atlanta) residents were emotionally bound to their city hospital patients for the intellectual satisfaction that they derived from medicine. When they entered practice they learned to treat private patients because their livelihood depended on it, but they always felt that they were being cheated by the patients. The patients did not have the right complaints and diseases. There were too few bumps and tumors, not enough coma and meningitis. There were too many headaches and too much indigestion. Duke offered the unusual opportunity of having the students, housestaff and junior staff take part in the care of private patients in a research and teaching setting. One could learn to combine the intellectual and emotional excitement of medicine with the creation of income. Furthermore, the public wards were only partly filled with the critically ill. Here was an opportunity to have an open admission policy, to admit anyone who felt they needed medical services. Here we could train residents to take care of sick people without the limitations of the artificial selection that is unavoidable in any crowded city hospital. Our aim was to free the doctor so that he could gain satisfaction from any health problem, and to create an atmosphere in which any patient would be a good subject for teaching. We have not always succeeded, but our students and staff have more freedom than most in these areas.

In training residents over a period of years, we have been impressed with the predictability of the behavior of a given resident in a given situation that involves interactions between people. We see the same resident become involved in the same way with each anxious family. Limited by his own reaction, he wastes a great deal of time and energy but seems to learn little from the experience. Observation shows that he is so bound by his own heredity, culture and education that he is not free to make a choice regarding his behavior. We have tried to give our staff the opportunity to develop more choice in their behavior pattern. Dr. Bingham Dai,[7] a member of the departments of Psychology and Psychiatry, worked with our two chief residents in the Department of Medicine each year. The work with Dr. Dai was on a voluntary basis yet all but two chief residents entered this program. Dr. Dai was paid by the Department of Medicine for his part in this program. The approach was psychoanalytic, and Dr. Dai determined the number of interviews and the duration of the process. The usual duration was one year. The department received no report or information of any kind except the bill.

These chief residents did achieve some emotional freedom from Dr. Dai. In every case, their spouses believed that they benefited. I observed that they took better histories, were more aware of other people's problems, and had more fun teaching. They enjoyed seeing all patients, and were very helpful in caring for patients whose problems were not described in the common medical texts.

Our third-year residents rotated through several clinical specialties. In the beginning they thought that they were profiting by the specific tool and techniques they acquired. As the year wore on and they had not used a tool for several months, we pointed out to them what this year was really about. They were learning how specialists work, what one has to do to become a

---

7. Bingham Dai was a Ph.D. psychologist in the Department of Psychiatry, Duke University Medical Center.

specialist, and how easy it was to acquire special knowledge. We gave them this experience with the idea of increasing their clinical freedom. In their careers—whether in practice, teaching or research—the need will inevitably arise for them to function in some areas for which they have not had special training. We wanted them to feel free to get the needed training and not to be bound by fear of the unknown.

Dr. Handler[8] and I commented some time ago on the fact that in the laboratory we also see "bound" students. They approach each problem with the tools they used in their first research efforts. They have a research tool in search of a disease. Learning new methodology is not difficult but they have had no experiences which showed them ease in which new skills can be acquired. In an effort to train students who will be more flexible in this area, the Duke medical school has set up a program to give selected students at any stage beyond the second year a year of investigative training. The clinician in this program will be an internist. In addition to advanced seminars and course work, these students will work on problems specifically designed to cross standard departmental lines. We hope the actual crossing of these lines will create a new feeling of freedom in the young scientist. This program was sponsored by a grant from the Markle Foundation, and its faculty paid by a grant from the Commonwealth Fund.

We have also been interested in the training of staff members. We have used three devices to encourage their interest in teaching. First, we have given status to teaching in the department. I have always been willing to do more than my share and have obviously enjoyed it. Second, we have had enough enthusi-

---

8. Phillip Handler, Ph.D., was Chair of Biochemistry at Duke from 1950 to 1969 and President of the National Academy of Science from 1969 to 1981.

astic and capable elder teachers to set a high standard of performance for the youngsters to meet. Lastly, we have allowed junior staff members to have complete responsibility in limited areas where everyone would give them credit for either success or failure. We have a purpose, also, in rotating the responsibility for introductory medicine. Jack Myers, John Hickham, Ted Schwartz[9] and Herb Sieker[10] have had this assignment in the last ten years. These men all went on to have distinguished careers in medicine.

We have been fortunate in having areas in the VA hospitals where relatively complete independence could be given. Jack Myers was the first chief of medicine at the Atlanta VA Hospital, and he took over the chairmanship of the medical department in Pittsburgh. Jim Warren was first chief of medicine in the Durham VA Hospital and then moved to Texas as departmental chairman.

Because we have given our staff the security that comes with leadership and performance, our staff have gained confidence. They have been confident of their ability and convinced that they could make departments and schools grow.

The central theme of our teaching program has been "to make students and trainees free." We have striven to make young physicians in training grow up with increased intellectual, emotional and professional freedom.

Having now graduated my first class of professors, I must face the future. Statistically, the future is not bright. All departments run downhill in the last part of the chairman's tenure. Why?

---

9. Ted Schwartz, M.D., was Chair and Professor of Medicine at University of Chicago, Presbyterian Hospital.

10. Herbert Sieker, is now retired and was for many years an outstanding pulmonary physician-scientist and clinician at Duke.

The answer lies in the fact that the scientific and educational needs of the department change with time. Intellectually, the chairman knows this, but it is difficult to make the necessary changes. The dean is more concerned with departments where new chairman are being picked. He cannot believe that a department, now strong, can wither. He does not appreciate the urgency of the situation.

The Department of Medicine at Duke needs new capital for retooling its shop and for its necessary risk venture in the educational field. If the departmental structure can be reworked and the shop put in order, the department will continue to grow and to produce leadership in the fields of patient care, teaching and research.[11]

We wish to extend our existing system of joint appointment. We believe that teachers who work both in clinical and preclinical areas have the greatest usefulness in making new areas of specialized knowledge available to the average medical student. We would like to try our wings with joint teaching assignments in areas of the University other than the medical school. Our first move into new fields will probably be in the field of genetics. My own belief is that the genetic approach offers the opportunity for the preventive medicine of the future. Genetic backgrounds will determine the disease states that can be activated by the environment. Preventive medicine will modify the environment for the particular person to prevent the development of the unfavorable genetic possibilities.[12]

---

11. While this request was written in 1959, the issues remain current for all Departments of Medicine.

12. This emphasis on genetics presaged by 40 years the Human Genome Project, and the formation of the Institute for Genome Sciences and Policy at Duke in 2000.

Chapter 13
Building a School

The Duke University Medical School is Dr. Davison's School.[1,2] He was there before the buildings were built, before the books were bought for the library, before an administrative staff was assembled, and before a single faculty appointment was considered. On all of our walls under the paint, one finds inscribed, "Davison was here."

Under Dr. Davison's guidance the medical school grew into a community of scholars concerned with all phases of knowledge. He concerned himself with the practice of medicine in the state, the South, and the nation. He built an outstanding library. He operated a clinical center which has steadily grown until it has a worldwide reputation. He developed a system of private university clinics which bring a steady flow of visitors to Duke to study their operation. He spread pediatricians far and wide over the land and laid the basis for the development of a children's clinical center at Duke. He recognized the vitalizing impact of research upon the corporate body of the medical school, but properly pointed to its inordinate demands. There were no slaves or masters on his form sheet. Dr. Davison had the ability to delegate responsibility to others. He required a high level of performance, demanding of others the same standards of

1. Stead EA, Jr. Building a school. *Amer. J. Dis. Child.*, 124:343, 1972.
2. Wilburt C. Davison was the first Dean of Duke Medical School and established the first faculty of Duke University Medical Center.

excellence he had for himself. Under his guidance the school was not paternalistic. If a faculty member failed at Duke, the credit for the failure belonged to him and not to the dean. If a faculty member succeeded at Duke, the dean made it clear that the credit for the success belonged to the faculty member and not to the dean.

Dr. Davison separated his personal feelings from his responsibilities to the school. He did not hesitate to state his own adverse opinion of an individual. If his performance in the school was good, he supported him while disliking him. He was interested in assembling an outstanding faculty rather than a social club.

Dr. Davison operated informally. He was known to the faculty simply as "Dave." He did not depend on props for dignity. Coatless and tieless, he was always the Duke Medical School. He believed that no rules should ever be written down if it were possible to avoid doing so. Why limit the future by the vision of the past?

Dave always knew that good administration required a personal touch. Accomplishments of faculty members, wives, or children were acknowledged by a note from the dean. Every patient with any interest in Duke was visited by him. In truth, the man seemed to have eyes in the back of his head and ears everywhere.

As with all good administrators, his word was his bond. He carried a little notebook attached to his wallet. Once he agreed to a course, it was noted in the book. The matter was then as good as accomplished.

Chapter 14

The Essence of a Viable Medical Center

In the last few years I have worked as a paid consultant for several medical schools.[1] I have been struck by the academic paralysis that afflicts these schools. They are trying to operate complex medical centers on the basis of models created years ago by Harvard and Hopkins. These models attempt to preserve the fiction that in a complex society a medical center can be operated successfully by academicians interested only in scholarly achievement and that every member of the clinical departments shall be skilled in and practice science, teaching and patient care. In the clinical areas, academic advancement is restricted to those who continue to produce scientific papers of high quality. This means that care of the patient is not academically rewarding and that clinical care in the medical center is below that given in good private clinics. This reduces the income of the clinical services and the hospital. The doctors staying in the medical center and caring for the patients there are below the caliber of the doctors moving into the surrounding communities. The best clinicians leave the medical school, set up in practice around the medical school and, in the case of Hopkins and Harvard, use the same hospital as the university faculty. They create income greatly in excess of that paid to the university faculty and contribute

---

1. Stead EA, Jr. This was a memo sent to Dean William Anlyan and all department chairs at Duke on May 24, 1977.

no money to the medical center to support its teaching and research activities.

Duke created another model. It is now being followed by a number of schools. In the eyes of the next generation, the creation of the Duke model will be looked on as Duke's greatest achievement.

When Davison[2] arrived at Duke he found that he did not have enough money to support a distinguished basic science faculty and a distinguished clinical faculty. He elected to put the majority of his funds into the basic science faculty and to have the clinicians fend for themselves. As of this date, the majority of the clinical faculty receive only $2,500 per year from the endowment funds of the University. Davison elected not to have a separate faculty called clinical professors. He knew that everyone's best effort was required to float the ship and he wanted as few class distinctions as possible. Davison elected to support academically those clinicians primarily engaged in practice. He did not put a limit on their incomes, but they voluntarily taxed their incomes to allow the development of well-rounded teaching and research programs in their departments and to help build needed buildings. Dave knew that these clinicians would create incomes greater than those received by the basic scientists. He had no objections as long as they shared this income with the clinical departments. Once the funding of the clinical departments was off his back, he could turn his attention to the development of other areas. During my tenure as department chairman, the money given to the department by the Dean's office was one-third to one-fifth as large as the budgets received by my young protogés as they took over departments of medicine in other schools. I was surprised when I came to Duke to discover that

---

2. Wilburt C. Davison, the first Dean of Duke University Medical School.

the administrators of the hospital had the same power in the Executive Committee that I did. Each of us had one vote. It slowly dawned on me that Duke Hospital had to pay its bills and that every move that I made in graduate education, clinical research, or clinical teaching had repercussions throughout the entire medical center. I quickly joined up with Dave, and in departmental affairs, our administrator had as equal a voice as our distinguished scientists.

Dave[3] had a very simple rule. Every member of the medical center who was not easily replaceable was entitled to academic standing. An M.D. or Ph.D. was not the requirement. As the medical center grew more complex, I recognized that we had to have more specialized people in the Department of Medicine. We needed the best clinicians. They were not going to achieve this level of expertise unless they worked long hours. We needed the best clinical scientists. They were not going to achieve this level of expertise if they worked long hours in the clinic. I promoted some persons for outstanding clinical skills and some for outstanding scientific work. I did not try to cover up what I was doing by having our senior clinicians build up bibliographies by writing pot boilers. They were professors because they were better doctors than could be found in the communities and because they did their share of teaching.

During my tenure as chairman, I had to recruit physician scientists and clinicians. The identification and recruitment of physician scientists was not difficult. The identification and recruitment of clinicians who could teach and hold our patient following was much more difficult. The physician scientist had both a reasonable income and free time. The key clinicians sacrificed their free time and had to be satisfied by their love of Duke

---

3. Wilburt C. Davison, the first Dean of Duke University Medical School.

and their satisfaction from their association with a steady flow of bright young students. These clinicians stayed at Duke at considerably less income than their less capable peers practicing in the community.

I looked at the total output of our department. If our department produced less scholarly works than other departments of medicine the Dean had an obligation to replace me. If the department gave less than excellent clinical services, I should be replaced. If the teaching was inferior, I should be removed. In order to meet all the goals of an academic department and pay the monthly bills, I had to have a diversified faculty. I could not be bound by guidelines laid down by the scientists in the medical school who were not responsible for complex service units.

In Dave's day, the differences between departments was appreciated and no attempt was made to require all departments to follow the same rules. The day of the chairman of surgery is laid out quite differently from that of the chairman of medicine. I had much more direct student contact because I did not spend those long hours in the operating room that are a necessary part of the surgeon's day. The chairman of surgery was obligated to spend many hours in the operating room training his young staff, and these hours are not available for contact with a large number of medical students. For these reasons a chairman of medicine will win a popularity contest over an equally competent professor of surgery. Both are equally essential to the medical center. Dave recognized that doctors in many highly specialized areas would create an adequate income in a relatively short working day and would have the reserve energy to write up case reports and clinical studies. The general internist, pediatrician, and psychiatrist spend many more hours creating less income than the specialist. When these senior staff had done their teaching and spent the necessary time for their continuing education, there was no energy for paper writing. Yet without these dedicated clinicians the medical center will grind to a halt.

I would urge the medical school not to destroy Duke's model which has worked so well. This means that the department is required to put out as much scholarly research as other departments in outstanding medical schools. It allows him to promote the senior personnel responsible for essential services on the basis of their excellent practice and teaching. It avoids the sham that they are being promoted on the basis of their science.

In closing, I will point out that in none of the institutions that I have visited as a consultant could you find a senior internist, pediatrician, or psychiatrist after 4:30 p.m. The reward system was determined by the academicians and the essential services rendered by the faculty to keep the medical center viable were not recognized. These medical centers are becoming more and more poverty stricken. The departments of medicine, pediatrics, and psychiatry are supported by the department of surgery. The support is given grudgingly and everyone lives in genteel poverty.

Chapter 15

The Nature of Administration
in Academic Health Centers

I have enjoyed teaching, research, and the practice of medicine.[1] To carry out these functions efficiently, I had to assign a portion of my time to the structuring of an administrative framework which would allow me to spend the majority of my time in the areas of my chief interests, namely teaching, practice, and research. Over the years I learned a number of interesting things which I will share with you tonight.

One has to be at peace with reality and not spend energy in non-productive ways. Administration is a game that has a series of rules. In this sense it is like baseball. One has to touch first base before reaching second and third bases. If a player insists on running to third instead of first base, he will not be allowed to play. Energy spent in railing at the rules is usually wasted because the railer has no way to change the rules.

The greatest threat to a part-time administrator like myself is the fulltime person who does nothing but administrate. He has to fill his day with administrative activities and is happy enough to fill in any spare time with committee meetings. I am strongly committed to an excellent administrative support system for professional activities provided it functions as a support system.

---

1. Stead EA, Jr. The nature of administration in academic health centers, unpublished essay, 1977.

When administration becomes an end in itself and professional activity becomes the support system, productivity in education, research, and practice declines. My younger colleagues in their innocence assume that medical schools, research establishments, hospital and medical practices are managed rationally. They are continually frustrated because the observed behavior of these systems does not fit the model of rationality. They unsuccessfully search for evidence that their observations are at fault. Frustrated, they waste energy railing at a system they do not understand whose next move they cannot appreciate. The problem is that medical centers are not operated by that portion of the brain that uses calculus and solves differential equations. The more primitive parts of the cortex determine feeling and produce religions, the Spanish Inquisition, Ayatollah Khomeini and the Iranian revolution, love, hate, fear, envy, insecurity and happiness. Intellectual effort goes into rationalizing the irrational but actual rationality is never achieved.

Once you know the systems are operated irrationally, you can have considerable influence because you accept things as they are, spend energy usefully in using the system to meet your own irrational needs. The system is of course not fair. I have three children and each at an early age told their parents that "It is not fair." Our only comment was "Yes; we know it." All administrators routinely use certain ploys and you should be familiar with them. Any request outside the accepted framework which requires administrative action is usually accepted in a way that leads one to believe action will occur. The administrator then does nothing. He knows that most requests are made on the spur of the moment, are not carefully thought out and are not of much importance to the one requesting the action. In the majority of instances, inaction solves the problem. I have felt sorry for my administrative colleagues because I always establish an agreed-upon time for a follow-up call. I note this on my calendar and the administrator eventually has to come through or admit that he has rejected the request.

The chairman of a department agrees that your request is very reasonable and that he would implement it but for the fact that the dean or vice-provost has established a firm policy preventing such actions. The amateur accepts this in good faith but the more experienced person inquires of the dean and finds out that he has established no such policy. This ploy is considered kosher and is played at all levels. The vice president invents preventive policies for the president and the president for the board of trustees. An effective chairman will make an excellent presentation of programs initiated by members of his department when he strongly supports them. The faculty member initiating a proposal will make a more effective presentation than the chairman when the proposal is of little interest to the chairman. In the latter situation, the chairman should step aside and urge direct communication with the executive committee and the dean. This serves several purposes. The faculty member has a better chance of his proposal being accepted. If it is rejected he is less paranoid.

Be wary of persons who will die for too many things. If you will die for nothing you are worthless. If each decision involves commitment to an unyielding principle and there is a large series of unyielding principles, you are useless. I vividly recall a faculty member who stood on the principle of always being right. Our architect had put a post in a place where it should not have been placed. My associate bloodied his nose every morning because by right the post shouldn't have been there. I walked around the post and each morning remembered that this error would be eliminated in our next construction. In playing the administrative game one learns the problems of specialization. A generalist can always be busy but the specialist is impotent when demand for his special services slackens. I learned the lesson first in regard to optimal use of clinical space. In Atlanta patients were separated by age, sex, and clinical specialty. On top of this they were separated by race. Some units overflowed, others were half empty. Personnel assigned to a particular area performed less effectively when they were shifted temporarily to other units.

In structuring my own administrative support system, I was taught again the same lesson I had learned from specialized space. An executive secretary who understands your work, meets the public effectively, types accurately, manages the files, and can pick up quickly the train of thought after each interruption is invaluable. A person dependent on others for each of these functions is less useful. The support system for the too-specialized chief office worker will likely be overspecialized and less productive. The ability to identify, and keep happy, productive persons in your organization determines the ceiling on your performance. The head of the unit must enjoy his work and let others know that he enjoys it. The secret of success lies in finding the right person for each job and establishing working conditions that allow each person to develop fully their potential but as yet unexpressed abilities.

Chapter 16

The Role of the University in Graduate Training

There is little to say about the past. Universities have, in general, not assumed the responsibility for the graduate training of physicians.[1] When the university has taken any responsibility, it has done so for a very restricted group of students. We can therefore discard the past and look toward the future.

Originally, there was little stimulus for the university to concern itself with medical graduate education. The training was hospital-oriented and concerned itself primarily with teaching the young physician to give health services by working as an apprentice to experienced physicians. It involved no contacts with the university departments of engineering, mathematics, business administration, information sciences, law, sociology, or political science. It related only slightly to the preclinical bioscientists on the faculty of the medical school.

Today, the scene is quite different. Medical centers are a much more integral part of the university, and the medical center could serve as a university-wide laboratory for physicians, bioscientists, engineers, sociologists, economists, lawyers, information scientists, and experts in business administration. No university has attempted to develop the full potential of its medical

---

1. Stead EA, Jr. The role of the university in graduate training. *Journal of Medical Education*, 44:739-744, 1969.

center. The purpose of this chapter is to draw attention to the advantages that will accrue to the entire university if it enlarges its role in medical graduate education. It can be accepted as a truism that the university will never enlarge its stake in medical graduate education until the university believes it will profit thereby.

The most intelligent use of university facilities for under-graduate and graduate medical educational purposes will never be possible as long as college, undergraduate medical school, internship and residency, service in the armed forces, and the continuing education of the physician are considered as separate packages. Many requirements which seem sensible when they are examined by the people responsible for a single one of these 5 packages can be seen to be ridiculous when they are examined as a single unit. Let us review the twelve to sixteen years which usually elapse between completion of high school and entry of the physician into practice.

When one appreciates the long span of time, it becomes obvious that the material memorized in the early years and not constantly used has little relevance to the actual practice of medi-cine. Most of the things memorized in the early years will be forgotten before the physician enters practice, and many of the painfully memorized theoretical concepts will have been discov-ered to be ill-founded.

Purposes of Medical Education

The long educational period for the physician has 4 purpos-es: (a) general education to make him a useful citizen; (b) lan-guage preparation to allow him to read the wide variety of books pertinent to biology and medicine; (c) problem-solving training to bring out his need to extend his reading ability, his need to learn additional language and to extend the usefulness of his central system of knowledge by increasing the number of connections; and (d) apprentice training to teach him the best use of present knowledge to improve health.

Language Ability

Ability to read and understand books is the most important function of education. Practice of medicine can be carried out if the student has a thorough knowledge of the English language and a working knowledge of the symbolic languages of mathematics, physics, and chemistry as they are now taught in high school or the first year of college. If he wishes to become a medical scientist, he will have to master a greater range of symbolic language. The emphasis should be placed on the ability to use symbolic language rather than on content. New content can be added at any time as needed if the ability to read is present. The student should have an agreed period of time in residence in the university as a substitute for the present system which requires that he complete his college work before he enters medical school and that he complete medical school before he starts his graduate work. Some progress is being made in this area. Colleges, by giving advanced credit for portions of high school work, are allowing a wider selection of material which can be included in the college years. Medical schools are slowly beginning to allow some freshman course credits for work already performed in college. Ideally, the student should be able to enter medical school whenever he has obtained the language to read the books required by work to be taken in medical school. Having met the language requirements, he could postpone learning new areas of content until they gain relevance to his career. Many a man has marked time in college in his third or fourth years, using up years which he would dearly like to have at a more meaningful time in his program of development. By making the time of college and medical school a continuum, one could introduce great flexibility into the system. This would not require the college to be under the medical school jurisdiction. Administratively, it probably would require the university to establish an agreed-upon division of tuition charges and an agreed-upon number of years to obtain the M.D. degree. This same approach of molding the segments into a whole would pay great dividends at the internship and residency levels. Many things can be left out of the undergraduate program to be picked up as needed in the graduate years. Some specialized knowledge can be learned early and used to help finance the years of residency training. The crossover points between various areas of specialty training become more diversified and productive when the entire time of undergraduate and graduate years is available.

Military Service

For the foreseeable future, the Army, Navy, Air Force, and Public Health Service will require that physicians give two years of their lives to the service of their country.[1] These years should be incorporated into the educational program. As matters now stand, many assignments in the service will be nonproductive for the physician. The medical schools must carry part of the responsibility for this failure. We have not supplied the country with an effective corps of supporting personnel to help the physicians. The armed forces have taken the lead in that direction. We have not established patterns of training in our own medical centers that demonstrate effective replacement of the physician in those areas where less skilled personnel can be effective. The basic diffi-

---

1. This essay was written at a time when military service was still mandatory.

culty lies in the fact that we have simply hoped that the need for two years of compulsory military service would disappear. Once we have accepted it as a part of our educational program, we can help both ourselves and the armed forces.

The Continuum

Postgraduate education has been carried on as a separate function. If one year of the residency were eliminated, the physician would have one day of each week for seven years which he could devote to continuing education with no loss of time. During these seven years, he can give an immense amount of medical service; develop his own office, home, and hospital health team; and establish a firm base of financial support. In addition, he will have made a permanent commitment to continuing education.

This approach to handing the problem as a unit will be effective if four principles are accepted:

1. Years under university supervision be substituted for the present requirements regulated by the college, the medical school, the armed forces, and the specialty boards.
2. No course work is taken without adequate language preparation.
3. Any subject can be omitted as long as the time normally used by that subject is also omitted.
4. The student is enrolled in the university on a lifetime basis and can return for further work at any time.

Any program involving the residency will not be significant unless it is planned on the scope described above. That program will produce a product having the flexibility to adapt profitably to our changing times.

The program described to date will, of necessity, be operated by academic faculty devoted to improvement of health services by creation of new knowledge in biology. Bioscience will be the area used for teaching problem-solving, even though it is recognized that there is no close coupling between the content of the biosciences and the practice of medicine. This is the correct focus for the university, traditionally more concerned with the future than with the present. It produces an excellent product, and with it lies our hope for truly revolutionary advances in the prevention and treatment of disease. Every state needs at least one medical school adequately supported to allow it to engage in health-related research and to produce its full quota of physicians with a primary orientation toward the problems of human biology.

In recent years, medical schools have been urged to widen their intake and admit students who have developed strong interests in sociology, industrial engineering, information sciences, business administration, psychology, economics, and political science. Schools have done this to a limited degree, but they have required the student, regardless of his preparation, to pass the heavily biologically-oriented portion of our basic science years largely by memorizing. Some students with a limited background in science will want the traditional material, but it would be profitable to give them the language preparation first. When we consider the entire period devoted to educating the doctor as a continuum, time presents no problem. The logical solution for those who do not wish to master the additional language requirements of biosciences is to allow them to learn problem-solving from such disciplines as engineering, information sciences, law, economics, and business administration. The medical faculty as now constructed does not have enough scholars in the fields which have been of the greatest interest to the non-bioscience student to feel comfortable in allowing him to take a less biologically-oriented course through medical school. He is therefore forced into the common mold.

The Medical Center as a University Laboratory

Medical centers could be ideal laboratories for many university departments. The computer-based communication sciences, industrial and systems engineering, electrical engineering, economics, sociology, psychology, and business administration have an increasing stake in the health field. They can never be very useful to health unless they have a portion of their departments based in medical centers and are conducting research programs that involve mixing their graduate students with medical personnel. If they use the medical center as a laboratory, they will begin to change the thinking of medical students. This faculty could be used to open the gates to allow more medical students to enter each freshman class. We would begin to open up opportunities for people with managerial talent to enter medicine. This program could increase the output of the school.

Establishing new laboratories and their faculties in medical centers obviously requires additional space and money. If the hospital is used as a university laboratory, each faculty member added may require less new space than his biologically-oriented counterpart. Traditionally, these new faculty members have been oriented to larger classes and to a more diverse output than the present biologically-oriented medical school faculties.

Shorter Term Goals

Medical educational programs need more stopping-off points between high school and entry of the physician into practice. At each stopping-off point, the student should have gained new skills which he can convert into dollars. At present, medicine not only requires a large investment of capital by the student, but it requires the ability to see far into the future. This presents no problem to the student who is able to work for many years with the payoff being in the distant future. This presents no problem to students coming from families with a long educational history, but it will keep many bright persons from other portions of our culture from becoming physicians even if free scholarships are supplied. There should be a series of shorter-term goals that can be reached more quickly and beyond which a portion of the students do not pass.

The question of how to build stepping stones is a complex one; and to think about it rationally, one has to consider the purpose of the long educational programs that produce our present physician. The theoretical justifications for the present programs are:

1. Physicians have an unexcelled opportunity to influence opinions of people who have major executive, legislative and judicial functions in shaping our society. For this reason, physicians should have broad background of knowledge concerning the origin and growth of our culture. They need an appreciation of evolutionary forces as they affect biology, social structures, and our physical world.

2. Physicians must, in the course of their daily work, make decisions that involve life and death. These decisions are important enough to justify a long educational experience.

3. Physicians use current knowledge and technology to take care of patients, but the rate of growth in technology and knowledge is so great that the physician must be continually changing over the years. Shorter, apprentice-based training will allow him to function well at the level of today, but this type of training will leave him further behind with each passing

year.

4. Advanced knowledge from all fields of basic science must eventually be applied to patients by physicians. Therefore, physicians must be trained, in part, as scientists if they are to be able to carry out this transfer function effectively.

These appear to me to be valid reasons for requiring the physician to have a long and varied education. As long as the physician gave the complete range of health services, there was no way to build in steps and keep the same quality of physician. He had to have all the education and training before he did anything. If society wishes to change the system, it has two alternatives: (a) eliminate a large part of the general education of the physician or (b) have places where he can effectively work without completing the entire program. If the physician remains responsible for the quality of the medical services but actually delivers some of the services through a variety of intermediates trained by the universities and medical centers, steps become possible as well as desirable. The absence of steps, each of which requires increased competence and each of which increases income, is currently the greatest block to bringing bright persons from poor families into medicine.

The Duke Curriculum

The Duke curriculum is well-adapted to steps. In Year 1 of the medical school, one has a survey of the basic sciences that underlie the practice of medicine. At the end of Year 1, the students are well-prepared to stop off and work in any area of the hospital, community, or health department laboratories. They can teach biological sciences in the high school or work in industrial pharmaceutical laboratories. They can work up through administrative programs that relate to science and medicine. Students spend Year 2 as clinical clerks in the hospital contributing to the care of the sick. They have the option to complete Year 2 eighteen months after they enter medical school. At the end of Year 2, they are prepared to serve as a clinical assistants to any physician or group of physicians. They can continue in basic science with a knowledge of the culture of health care and the potential tragedy of living and dying.

The Apprenticeship

It would be possible to increase the number of steps between high school and the physician's entering practice by making use of a combination of apprentice and non-apprentice training. As noted previously, apprentice training is effective in teaching the best medicine of today. It fails in producing the best medicine for tomorrow. Students from high school and on can be taught medicine effectively by the apprentice approach. On the basis of the performance of today, they will not be distinguishable from our present physicians. They would make ideal assistants but not leaders. At the end of two years of apprentice training, one could select the students who have the ability to become complete physicians and give them the necessary general and scientific education to reach that goal. Throughout the rest of their education, they could continue to give some service and create some income.

Summary

The fragmentation of twelve to sixteen years of training between at least 5 agencies will always result in chaos. The next great advance in medical education will come when one or more universities assume responsibility for the lifelong education of the physician.

Chapter 17

The Setting of the Hanes Ward Project

F or many years doctors have given lectures to nurses and nurses have helped doctors care for patients.[1] In spite of these areas of close contact, the pattern of education in the medical schools and in the nursing schools developed along different lines. The nursing educators paid less attention to patient care and to the problems arising from patient care. They turned these areas over to nursing service — a separate organization under control of the hospital — and concerned themselves primarily with educational theory and didactic instruction. While nursing instructors taught certain practical aspects of nursing in the hospital, they carried no responsibility for the welfare of the patient. By contrast, the medical school closely integrated patient care and teaching. The chief of the medical service in the hospital is the chairman of the Department of Medicine; the chief of the surgical service is the chairman of the Department of Surgery. Students and residents care for patients as they learn clinical medicine.

The faculty in nursing stressed the need for advanced degrees. These were usually taken in education or one of the

---

1. Stead EA, Jr. The setting of the Hanes Ward Project, unpublished essay. February 1963. In 1963, a major part of the medical service at Duke was on the ward named after the second Chair of Medicine at Duke, Frederic M. Hanes, M.D.

social sciences. The net effect of this was that the members of the nursing faculty were usually less competent in dealing with sick patients than the average nurse. The more advanced the degree, the less capable one became of adding excitement to the clinical service.

The doctor felt that his education program was the most desirable. The nursing faculty felt that they had escaped the hospital burden. In the pressure of busy days, there was little opportunity for the doctors and nurses to watch each other teach and to exchange ideas. One obvious solution to the communication problem was to have a senior faculty member of one school work for a time as a member of the faculty of the other school. The question was, who? I, as the chairman of the Department of Medicine, was at that time a member of the nursing advisory council. I was impressed with the ability of Miss Thelma Ingles, who was the member of the nursing faculty responsible for the teaching of the courses in medical and surgical nursing. I watched her teach and observed the response of the students to her method of bedside teaching, a technique rarely used effectively in the nursing school. I felt that Miss Ingles had the ability to teach both the theoretical aspects and practical aspects of nursing at the same time and that, with some additional studies in clinical physiology, she would be an even more effective bedside teacher.

One day at an advisory council meeting Miss Ingles announced that she would be away from Duke for her sabbatical year. I suggested that she join the Department of Medicine for a year and find out how much of the philosophy of clinical teaching in the medical school was applicable to teaching for nursing. I offered to reserve the afternoon hours of 5 to 6 three times weekly for discussion of patients, clinical physiology, teaching and administration. In addition, I would arrange for special instruction in any of the clinical areas which Miss

Ingles wished to explore. Miss Ingles did spend a year in this way.

The educational experiences centered about problems that arose from the care of patients on the medical service of Duke Hospital. It became obvious that there was a large body of knowledge that was very useful to a nurse which was nowhere included in either undergraduate or graduate nursing education. Would it not be possible to give an advanced degree in nursing that would really signify increased competence in nursing itself? Would not more understanding of the clinical physiology and pathology underlying the behavior of the ill patient allow the nurse to assume more responsibility? Could not such a nurse be given more flexible assignments? Could she not determine without specific orders whether to follow a set routine or to modify the routine to fit the specific problem?

By mid-year, Miss Ingles and I were convinced that a master's degree based on study of patients was possible, and in the last half of the year Miss Ingles began to reduce these ideas to written form. A master's program designed to give greater competence in nursing was approved by the University and a grant from the Rockefeller Foundation underwrote the first years of the program.

In the master's program, Miss Ingles worked closely with Morton Bogdonoff,[2] from Medicine, and faculty from the departments of Psychiatry and Sociology. The nurses centered their learning around problems presented by patients. They read relevant material from psychiatry, physiology, medicine and sociology and discussed the subject matter among themselves and with their faculty advisors. They worked closely with the physicians. They observed the impact of the dietitian, physiotherapist,

---

2. Morton Bogdonoff was a faculty member in the Department of Medicine from 1957 to 1970.

occupational therapist and ward nurse on the patient. They learned the specialized procedures necessary for good nursing care in severe complicated illness. They also learned to care for the anxious, complaining patient who did not require complicated mechanical devices to maintain life.

While the master's program was developing, Miss Ingles had started a more active training program in the medical clinic. Nursing students were working with medical students, interns and resident in the care of the patients. The nurse in charge of the nursing students worked closely with Dr. Bogdonoff, who was responsible for the medical care of the patients and the teaching of medical students, interns and residents. These joint teaching experiences were enjoyed by the members of the medical faculty and nursing faculty.

As an outgrowth of these experiences, the program in medical nursing for seniors was modified to include more opportunities for learning at the bedside. Senior students assigned to individual patients gave nursing care under a three-member team that included a junior staff member, each from Medicine and Psychiatry. The senior students enjoyed their experiences and perceived that they were receiving many satisfactions from their nursing experiences that were not shared by the nurses working in the hospital. They appreciated that hospital nursing the country over was organized on the basis of making do with as few nurses as possible. They believed that as graduate nurses they would never have a chance to practice the type of nursing they had been taught.

During the winter months a group of the senior students discussed with Miss Ingles the possibility of nursing in an area in the hospital under the guidance of the nursing faculty. They wished to have enough nurses in this areas to nurse in the manner learned in the nursing school. They finally instructed their leaders to learn from me whether the medical department would be interested in their nursing Hanes ward. If there was interest, they requested that Miss Ingles and I work out this program with the hospital.

The students emphasized that they did not wish to change the ward into an intensive nursing unit. They wished to nurse the acutely ill, the moderately ill and the ambulatory patients. They wanted the composition of the ward to be unchanged. They were as interested in the anxious ambulatory patient as they were in the patient desperately ill with chronic lung disease. They did not wish the patients to be transferred to other wards as they improved. They wanted the same nurses to care for the patient during serious illness and during convalescence. They wanted to staff the ward so that private-duty nurses would not be needed. They had no objection to an extra nursing charge for anyone who came on the ward, because they believed that additional nursing service would justify the charge.

The Department of Medicine was glad to help with this project. A committee with representatives from Medicine, nursing service, nursing school and the hospital was set up to work out the administrative details. The plan was opposed by the head of the nursing service for two main reasons: (1) the concentration of nurses on a ward with only an average number of sick persons was indefensible and would adversely affect nursing morale throughout the entire nursing service; and (2) all nursing procedures throughout the hospital had to be the same and could not be modified at the ward level even by an experienced faculty member. Miss Ingles and I were insistent that a member of the nursing faculty be in charge and that she have the power to change assignments of time and procedures as needed. I believed that the program should be supported by patient fees and that a charge should be made which would not only support the additional nurses in the unit but would create some funds to support a clinical nursing faculty. I projected a clinical nursing faculty with members and incomes beyond those usually supplied by universities or hospitals, and believed that this projection was realistic if Duke became known as a place where exceptional nursing was available. I believed that the income created should be handled by a business manager selected by the nursing school and that the nurses working on the ward should be responsible to the nursing school and to the hospital. The chief hospital administrator at the time did not wish to change the traditional pattern of relationship between the nurses and the hospital. He wanted the funds created to go into the general budget and all employment to be handled through his office.

As might be guessed, these issues were settled by compromises. The administrators agreed to the program, provided it was projected primarily as an educational program. In addition to their regular ward work, the Hanes nurses would take work in the graduate school giving them an agreed-upon number of hours of credit towards a master's degree. An administrative chart was drawn up which shared responsibility between nursing service and nursing school. Funds created by the surcharges on Hanes were kept in a separate account and monies created above added cost went into a fund under control of a committee with representatives from nursing school, nursing service, hospital administration, and the Department of Medicine.

Hanes Ward was very successful. Nursing was headed by Ruby Wilson, a rising young star in the area of medical and surgical nursing. The ward was staffed by graduates of Duke Nursing School. Morale was high and the young nurses were working long and rewarding hours.

The Ward created a profit from day one, no other unit in the state could compete in terms of patient satisfaction. The first signs of trouble occurred when the administration refused to purchase an extra coffee pot for some of the informal sessions between the nurses and the ambulatory patients. Were not the profits of the venture to accrue to the Hanes project and not to the general budget?

The Hanes nurses had worked longer and harder than the usual staff nurses. In those days acute admissions were rare the week before Christmas. The Hanes ward would be filled with chronic patients requiring custodial rather than skilled nursing care. I offered to cover Hanes ward by employing a number of my patients who could give custodial care and allow the nurses a Christmas break. The administration was adamant: No Christmas breaks for Hanes nurses. The final break came in the late spring when the head of nursing services, Miss Clark, and the Hospital administration, Mr. Frenzel, refused to release the profit made by the Hanes nurses to the nursing school. The project ended at the end of 12 months. All of the Hanes staff resigned and none of the graduating nursing class applied to Duke Hospital. The bad feelings created never subsided and eventually ended in the closure of the Duke nursing school. Doctors in the medical school closed the nursing school when they felt that the output of the school was no long a support system for patient care in Duke Hospital.

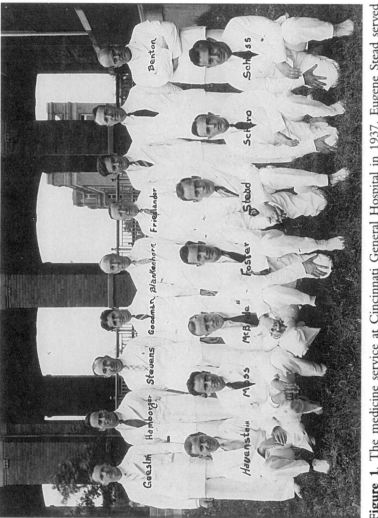

Figure 1. The medicine service at Cincinnati General Hospital in 1937. Eugene Stead served six months as an assistant resident and 12 months as chief resident (first row, third from the right).

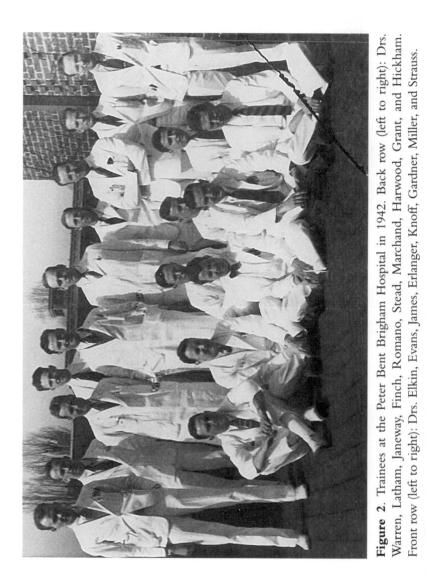

Figure 2. Trainees at the Peter Bent Brigham Hospital in 1942. Back row (left to right): Drs. Warren, Latham, Janeway, Finch, Romano, Stead, Marchand, Harwood, Grant, and Hickham. Front row (left to right): Drs. Elkin, Evans, James, Erlanger, Knoff, Gardner, Miller, and Strauss.

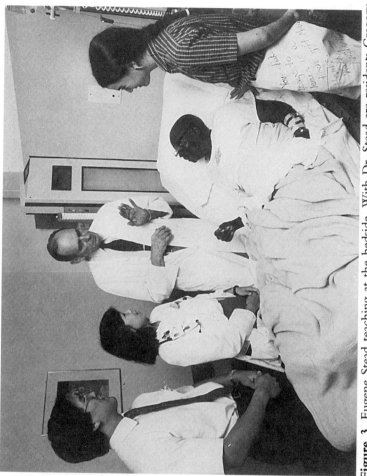

Figure 3. Eugene Stead teaching at the bedside. With Dr. Stead are residents Gregory Chow, Severana Chen, and Kathy Merritt.

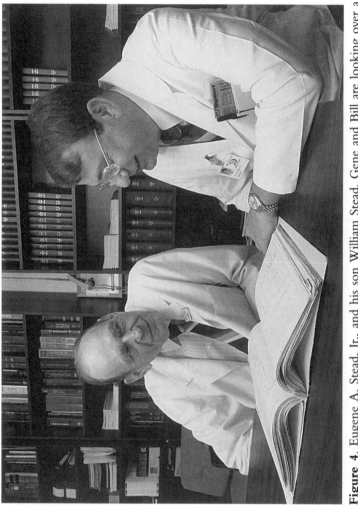

Figure 4. Eugene A. Stead, Jr., and his son William Stead. Gene and Bill are looking over a paper medical record. Their collaboration over the years would set the stage for electronic health information systems at both Duke and Vanderbilt Medical Centers.

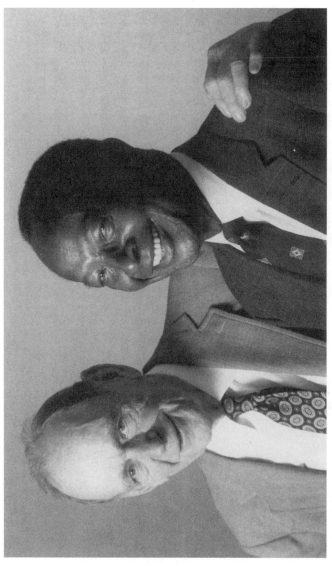

Figure 5. Eugene A. Stead, Jr., with Charles Johnson, M.D. (right). Dr. Johnson was the first African American physician hired at Duke. Dr. Stead recruited Dr. Johnson to Duke from his practice at Lincoln Hospital in 1970. Dr. Johnson, a former president of the National Medical Association, was a mainstay on the clinical service at Duke in the Division of Endocrinology until his retirement in 1996.

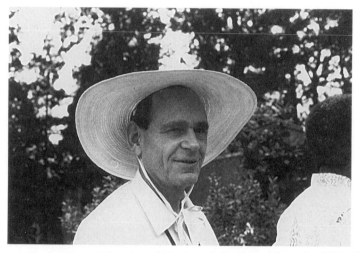

Figure 6a-b. Gene (above) and Evelyn (below) in China in 1973. This was one of the most exciting trips the Steads took and provided Gene with ideas about new ways for healthcare systems to work.

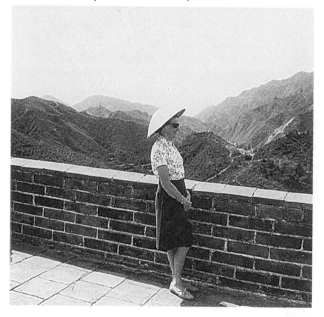

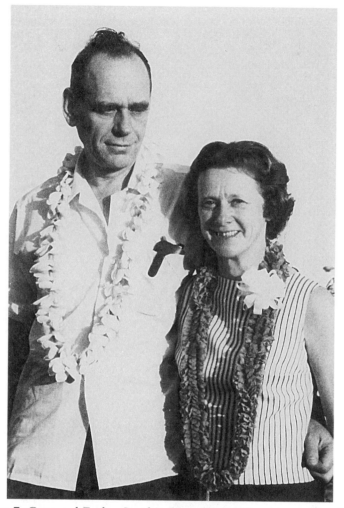

Figure 7. Gene and Evelyn Stead in Hawaii in 1968, one year after Gene retired from the Chair of Medicine job at Duke.

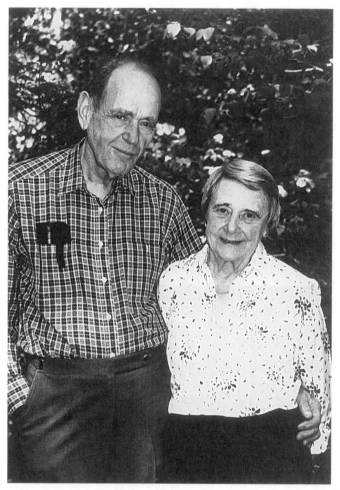

Figure 8. Gene and Evelyn in April 1995 at their home in Bullock, North Carolina.

III

The Computerized Medical Database: The Way of the Future

D uke University is interested in developing the Duke Medical Center and its community-based health science ventures as a laboratory for the University, where the departments of Economics, Mathematics, Information Sciences, Systems Engineering, Business and Sociology can work in the real world. We are establishing new relationships with the undergraduate and graduate faculties of the University which will result in members of the departments listed above having a greater influence on the medical school's admission policy and curriculum. The medical school intends to enlarge the intellectual base on which clinical training is given.

Chapter 18

Creation of Personnel at the Medical/ Computer Science Interface: Should It Be a Specialty?

The development of minicomputers and microprocessors allows the paper and pencil records to be replaced by electronic records.[1] Data from medical practice stored in paper form disappear in office files and hospital record rooms. Only a fraction are retrieved for retrospective studies. Records kept in electronic form are immediately available and over time give the doctor a database from which he can construct a computerized textbook describing his own practice in terms of diagnosis, treatment and outcomes. The data from the practice are available as a basis for clinical trials of drugs and procedures. The doctor has a database for biostatistical and epidemiologic studies relating to his practice.

To bring the electronic age to the practice of medicine, we need to produce a new breed of practicing doctors with a basic science experience in signal processing, computer programming, bioengineering, biostatistics, and epidemiology. During the maturation of practicing doctors, they needs two years of fellowship experience in areas of clinical practice that use the material they

1. Stead EA, Jr. Creation of personnel at the medical/computer science interface: Should it be a specialty? *Journal of Medical Systems*, 8:3-6, 1984.

have learned in the information sciences undergirding medical computing.

What name is suitable for these emerging clinical specialists? We can add a qualifying clause to any of the existing specialists: family practitioner-clinical information specialist, orthopedist-clinical information specialist, general internist-clinical information specialist. Another possible title is clinical information scientist.

The term *clinical information* covers a broad area. One usually turns to the library for medical information. It is at present stored in books, journals, cassettes and tapes. The portion of the library information system that is useful in clinical practice was obtained from observations on patients. The majority of the material has been generated from retrospective studies of office or hospital records. A small portion of the material comes from prospective studies performed in a research mode and financed by the National Institutes of Health, other governmental agencies, or by the pharmaceutical industry.

The advent of minicomputers, word processors and microprocessors has provided the machinery for a new type of record keeping which makes it possible to process, store, analyze and use the information from everyday practice in a way that was not possible in the past. We are just beginning to see a change in the evaluation of the quality of medical practice. Evaluation of quality by determining the degree to which recommended processes are followed is giving way to evaluation of quality by outcomes. The electronic record will give doctors in practice a stake in using information and in adding to the store of information.

Combining medical information and accounting into a single interactive system produces an error-free system that controls all functions generating charges. Accountants keep accurate books with voluminous volumes of paper on charges that reach their system. In our work as consultants to medical practices in medical centers, we are impressed again and again with the money lost before the accountant enters the picture. Charges not made, charges lost, charges destroyed, or charges made late are more costly than the cost of an integrated medical and financial computerized system.

In the interactive system, the charge is an integral part of the performance of a service. Entry of an order generates a requisition in the service department and a charge in the accounting record. If a service unit does not perform procedures without a requisition, no charges are lost or late. The interactive system performs internal control functions. Reports to the service departments can be limited to summary trend data which give the numbers and types of different procedures performed and allow effective management of scarce resources.

The push for an interactive medical and business accounting system will have to come from doctors steeped in the culture of medicine who are aware of the many slips and errors that cause conventional systems to create financial losses. The accountants blissfully using the computer as an adding machine will testify that they have checked the addition and verified the accuracy of the computing. Being unaware of where the losses are occurring, and having no experience with interactive systems, the accountants cannot induce change. They can and will produce passive resistance to change.

In my day, to graduate from high school one had to spell correctly and write an acceptable English theme to move into upper class status at college. Today, colleges are requiring computer literacy before entering the third year and additional computer skills before entering graduate schools. Our entering medical students now use computers as my generation used typewriters and slide rules.

We can anticipate that in the near future the doctor entering practice will be prepared to computerize the management of the business aspects of his office and to have at his disposal enough computer power to handle his medical records. In most instances he will not have learned to use this computer capacity in the daily practice of medicine. He will continue to rely on written records and will not record the medical data electronically where it would be easily accessible and available. Properly recorded and analyzed, the data from his practice could be used as his own textbook.

Persons skilled in medical practice and knowledgeable about computers, statistics, epidemiology and the ways to create and use medical data produced in daily practice are in short supply. Medical schools have not included information sciences in their curriculum and have not developed a faculty and student body for these areas. The impetus for the development of these clinical specialists comes from the clinical faculty in the medical schools and graduates of the schools who wish they were more competent in medical computing.

Our prediction is that in the near future a few medical schools will formalize programs in the curriculum allowing the person with a bioengineering degree to develop competence in medical computing at the medical undergraduate level and to extend this competence by two years of fellowship experience taken in conjunction with conventional residency programs. At Duke, the third-year student selects his courses from a menu of basic science offerings. Course work is available in signal processing, biostatistics, epidemiology, and ways to develop an interactive, integrated medical and financial information system. There are functioning clinical programs using computerized information systems in cardiology, neurology, cancer, nephrology, obstetrics, and psychiatry. The faculty in these units can identify clinical programs that give practical expression to the students of the theoretical concepts taught in the structured courses. In these laboratories the students learn to identify various ways of handling medical and accounting information and to identify areas where improvements must be made to meet the needs of diverse medical practices. Students taking this medical undergraduate information tract are to form the core of persons interested in becoming two-year fellows in the medical computing and information sciences.

The faculty for this specialty in private medical schools will be supported largely by funds from clinical departments, because it is at the practice interface where the largest number of these information specialists are needed. Some special arrangements are needed to supply faculty in those areas not usually covered by conventional medical school faculty. In theory, this could be handled by having a joint program where the medical school supports the M.D. and the engineering school supports the bioengineer. To be successful, this requires a bioengineer expert in computer science who believes enough in the venture to live with practicing doctors and serve as the communicator with other needed resources in the engineering and business schools. The coordinator of the program should be a practicing doctor who has worked collaboratively with bioengineers in the development of computing systems for use in medical practice. To be effective, bioengineers will have to be geographically located where doctors are practicing. They will have more medical undergraduate and graduate students than engineering candidates for the Ph.D. The engineering school may not wish to pay the salary of the bioengineer located outside their traditional areas of operation. They may prefer that the medical school finance the entire program, restricting the role of the engineering school to assuring the quality of the bioengineer employed by the medical school. Teaching one course in the engineering school and access to engineering graduate students is the best assurance of quality.

I stress the importance of clinicians having had active hands in the construction as well as in the use of systems for clinical practice because this experience will teach them the importance of a collegial relation with the bioengineers. A doctor who uses computer programs but has never worked side by side with his bioengineering colleague tends to treat the bioengineer as a technician. Programs useful for medical practice require careful evaluation of the doctor/computer interface. A change in the behavior of the doctor may be an easier solution to a new problem than a more expensive and time-consuming adaptation of the machine. The medical coordinator of the program needs to be able to handle a reasonable amount of formal course work and have a working knowledge of the clinical laboratories in the various divisions.

The program would be similar to the pattern already existing in other areas in most medical schools. The year in the medical school would be taught as a year in basic science. The apprentice aspects of the instruction essential to making the formal course work meaningful would be a function of the ongoing clinical laboratories engaged in procuring data and processing information. Two members of the faculty — the clinical coordinator and the bioengineer — would be paid by the program. The operating clinical laboratories would supply statisticians, epidemiologists, and accountants for the formal course work. Faculty members in these areas are already supported by funds outside the proposed program. They will be repaid for their efforts when fellows are available for two years of graduate work in clinical areas.

The time has come for those doctors who can qualify as clinical information specialists to define college, medical school and graduate experiences needed to produce clinical information specialists. The first step will be to organize a society for these specialists. The first goal of the society would be to modify the curriculum content of medical schools, residency and fellowship programs to give due credit for the courses and laboratory work in the area of clinical information. The second priority would be to find funds for faculty and fellows.

The funds for the program can come from endowed professorships, from industry, from foundations, or from line items identified in the budgets of state supported schools. Funds will not be found until leaders in the area of medical computing and information sciences define their educational objectives and describe in detail the requirements for undergraduate and graduate education.

Chapter 19

The Way of the Future

O ver the last ten years I have kept an eye on the possible role of technology and of a different mix of health professionals on the delivery of personal health services.[1] Seven years ago I decided that the day of technology had not arrived and I elected to diversify the manpower mix. This led to the development of the Duke physician's assistant or associate program. I never lost our interest in the machines, however, and today I believe their time has come. We are on the brink of a major technological breakthrough in the practice of complex medicine. This technological revolution will change the educational patterns in medical schools, will have far-reaching effects on patterns of practice in the medical centers, and will give the medical centers the leverage in community hospitals to set up a reasonable regionalization program.

Before proceeding with the main thesis, I must acknowledge that many prophets in the last two decades have predicted that technology would by 1972 already have swept the medical fields of education and practice. In actual fact, little change has occurred. At the practice interface, doctors have discovered that they need little information to practice medicine in the current modes. A list of the patient's problems (diagnoses), a summary of

---

1. Stead EA, Jr. The way of the future. *Trans. Assoc. of Amer. Phys.*, 85:1-5, 1972.

past diagnostic procedures, current medications, and a flowsheet of procedures to be done give them all the useful information that is easily available to them or to any of their colleagues. While this arrangement of the patient's record can be done with the computer, it can be made available to doctors in other cheaper and equally useful formats. Computer-aided instruction is available to them but journals, books, audiodigests, medical meetings and exchanges of information with colleagues offer equally effective routes of education. There is nothing offered by the new approaches that is worth the trouble of overturning well-formed, lifelong patterns of practice and learning.

My thesis is that major changes in medical education and practice will not occur until there is a practical demonstration that doctors or groups of doctors using computer technology have a clear advantage in practice over doctors who maintain the status quo. An important facet of practice that has no solution other than computerization has not as yet been defined. This presentation defines such a program and outlines a practical demonstration that could be in operation within a period of three years.

Doctors in the practice of medicine collect a wide variety of information which allows them to make diagnoses. A diagnosis puts a patient into a subgroup of the population which is supposed to have a common outcome if untreated. Medical care is useful if it can favorably modify the lives of patients who form this subgroup. The doctor may be useful if he determines that persons placed in a particular subgroup really do not have a common outcome. Many persons with a diagnosis of a potentially fatal illness can live a useful and unworried life if they can be informed that they are in a subgroup within the diagnostic category that does not have the morbidity and mortality characteristics usually associated with that particular diagnosis.

In actual practice, persons within a given diagnostic category (subgroup) may have widely different outcomes. A person with myocardial infarction may die in three minutes or live for 50-plus years. Doctors, therefore, on the basis of textbook and journal information and from their own experience, attempt to establish a few sub-categories under each diagnosis. The number they can carry in their head is small, and they are continually tricked by the capriciousness of their memory. If one watches them practice, one finds that the experiences of the last few months weigh unduly in their decision-making. One learns by experience that the behavior of doctors is not understandable unless the most recent inputs that affect their decision-making can be captured. Periodically they will be disturbed by their ignorance and, with great effort, will review the past experience of themselves and their colleagues to determine the best treatment of a patient 60 years or older who has diabetes, myocardial infarction and aortic stenosis. To their chagrin, they will discover that they have not established rigid criteria for any of the three diagnoses and that neither they nor their colleagues have the information vehicle that will allow them to determine whether patients they are studying are a relatively homogeneous group with a predictable outcome or are a very heterogeneous group with widely differing outcomes. Fully knowing that they do not have good information, but urged on by the stimulus to give the best care to the next patient they see with these diagnoses—and frequently by the desire to write a paper—they make the assumption that these patients are a tight subgroup and they proceed accordingly. They are neither better nor worse than any other doctor trying to describe the course of a chronic illness and endeavoring to give the patient good medical care.

An unusually compulsive doctor, collecting data on illnesses of short duration, will have better information on the course of the patients placed into a particular subgroup. But even here he is confronted with more subgroups than his memory can handle. He must deal with the disease from infancy to old age, from disease discovered early on the basis of symptoms to disease discovered by accident, from disease localized at discovery to disease generalized at discovery, from the process producing no disability to the process producing severe disability, from the disease producing no change beyond the first involved system to disease producing change in one or more than 20 subsystems, from disease occurring in very genetically different hosts. It must come as no surprise that, with the exception of very acute processes, doctors are poor predictors of the course of illness, with or without treatment.

Computer science can change this picture. Information can be collected and stored in a way that allows doctors to use all their experience to care for the patient—not just the portion they can remember. They can use the total experience of themselves and of their medical center, and eventually that of other medical centers, to care for their patients. The computer can carry more subgroups in its memory than can the doctor. Only an examination of outcomes can determine the number of useful subgroups.

The Duke Medical Center has for the last five years been collecting a computerized database to assist our doctors in caring for complex cardiovascular problems.[2] Our first problem was to develop a data management team composed of doctors and computer scientists who are willing to make an investment in establishing a data bank that any doctor in practice in our institution could use. This data management group has worked with experts in the cardiovascular field to define the descriptors to character-

---

2. Out of Dr. Stead's database grew the Duke Clinical Research Institute (DCRI), the largest not-for-profit clinical research organization in the world. The DCRI is now led by a Stead protégé, Dr. Robert Califf.

ize the individual patient. These descriptors are as close to the primary data as possible and are not a condensation of data into a conclusion or diagnosis. The statement that the changes in an electrocardiogram are diagnostic of myocardial infarction is not very helpful. A description of the electrocardiogram is much more useful. The primary data remain useful even if the criteria for the diagnosis of myocardial infarction change over time or with a new set of doctors. The descriptors of the patient population will, of course, change with experience. Many will be found to be useless. Medical science will demonstrate the need for new ones.

The data management team had to convince the doctors that the data collected from the patients belonged to the institution and not to them. This meant that there had to be agreement on definitions and that all the data had to be stored in a central file. The doctors had to give up their prerogative of storing parts of the data in their private files and changing the data whenever they felt that new information made their previous groupings erroneous. The doctors had to accept the fact that the data management section would not process data to build the bank unless it was validated and that, in many instances, non-physician personnel would be better validators than the doctors themselves.

The traditional functions of storing, clustering the data and retrieving the data have presented an interesting series of problems, but they are not nearly as difficult as the problems of collecting validated data for input into the system. Collection of a proper database cannot be piggy-backed onto practice. The creation of the database is expensive. The doctor in practice can use the database, and this expense can be borne by patient care funds. The development of the database and its extension by data from new patients is expensive, and every doctor using the database cannot contribute new data to the base.

The use of the database is based on the fact that we are

matching our patient with patients who are enough like him to have a similar course either treated or untreated. This means that both short-term and long-term outcomes must be known. This adds a new dimension to medical practice because the knowledge of outcomes of similar patients becomes an essential part of the data bank. This is an expensive but necessary part of the system.

We are now far enough along to begin to feel the power of the database in the daily practice of medicine. We intend to reach the point where no clinical decisions will be made on the care of any patient with coronary artery disease, myocardial infarction or heart block until the data bank has been searched and the outcomes of similar patients have been given to the doctor. When the Duke Medical Center can immediately bring all its experience to bear on each cardiovascular patient entering its doors, it will have a clear lead over all other doctors. It will be in the position of those departments of pathology that began to use electron, phase and fluorescent microscopy. Other pathologists hated to learn the new way but, to remain competitive, they had to use the new tools.

Once the problem has been cracked in a major area in a single medical center, progress will be rapid. Patient care funds will be a better financial resource, because the care given by the updaters and users of the data bank will be of superior quality. The greatest profits from the system will accrue when several medical centers begin to pool their data. At the present time there is not enough incentive for different medical centers to reach common definitions, common methods of validating data, and a common method for storage and retrieval. When one medical center has established the system, there will be a strong incentive for other centers to put their house in order and join the system. We are also pushed to implement an adequate system for describing and more accurately subgrouping patients by the amount of public money being expended to evaluate therapeutic procedures in chronic illness.

Patients with a common diagnosis are usually randomized into two groups—one treated and one not treated. The statisticians erroneously believe that patients with a given diagnosis are a homogeneous subgroup and, untreated, still have a common outcome. Nothing can be further from the truth. Patients given the diagnosis of coronary arterial disease are not a homogeneous group. No one knows how many subgroups would have to be defined to select persons who ran a reasonably common course. My own guess would be 100. No single institution can produce enough patients to define all the clinically useful subgroups. In desperation all the patients are considered to be alike and some therapeutic intervention is started. The intervention may cause great harm to some, not affect others, and help some. The study predictably comes out with no sharp answer except for the bill of many millions of dollars.

Chronic, multifactorial disease problems can be studied but not by the methods of the present or past. If one wishes to create useful information on which to base therapeutic trials, computer technology must be exploited.

When this system becomes operational, major changes will occur in medical education. The introduction into medicine will not be through anatomy or biochemistry. It will be through the information sciences as they are used in medicine. Duke Hospital Information System will become a resource available to hundreds of patients each day who never see Duke. It will allow easy monitoring of the reliability of the descriptors that are collected in all the communities in North Carolina and will give us the necessary feedback to develop a reasonable program of continuing education. It will allow, at both the medical center and the community level, continued exploration of the best use of all professional manpower.

The present emphasis in medical education is on diagnosis. The emphasis in the future will be on ways of collecting accurate descriptors of the patient. If these descriptors are varied enough and accurate enough, the doctor will search the database, not for a diagnosis but for patients whose descriptors correspond to those of his patient. He will know the outcomes of the treated and non-treated patients similar to his current patient, and he will be in a position to give the best care to his patient.

The program to change the medical information base on which the practice of medicine rests requires the active participation of computer scientists, medical investigators and active practitioners. It requires a place in the medical center where faculties of mathematics, computer science, bioengineering and medicine can work together. In such a facility, graduate students from these various disciplines can interact as they complete their education. The Duke Medical Center is fortunate in that the university departments of computer science and of bioengineering have established units in the Medical Center. We now have the capacity to staff the proposed program. Implementation of the program will increase the educational opportunities for graduate work in medical information systems.

In summary, major technological changes will not occur in medical schools until this technology can accomplish worthwhile results which give the practitioner using these tools an advantage over his competitors. Therapeutic trials in chronic illness cannot be meaningful until better ways to form tighter subgroups that run a uniform course are operational. It will not require elaborate programs to evaluate the success or failure of this program. If doctors not using the system can compete successfully with doctors using it, the program has failed. If successful, it will be as obvious as the success of penicillin treatment of pneumonia. If it is not obvious, there will be no need for a long complex evaluation that might end up in calling failure success.

Chapter 20

The National Library of Medicine: The Great Equalizer Between Small Hospitals and Major Medical Centers

P hysicians in outlying communities and administrators of small hospitals are worried that patients will drive by them to obtain services from doctors and hospitals in the larger cities.[1] Today's informed patients know that smaller cites and hospitals cannot afford extensive information centers on their premises. They want to go where doctors have access to the most up-to-date information.

To answer this need, the National Library of Medicine, in Bethesda, MD, has developed its services to the point that anyone with a personal computer (or PC) and a modem can have access to its extensive files cheaply and quickly. The rural practitioner can have the same information that is used by doctors at our best medical centers.

The National Library of Medicine has made a special effort to open its data files to non-librarians. The library's *Grateful Med*, a name that reflects a bit of bureaucratic whimsy, is remarkable not only for what it does but for its low price. It allows the staff of any hospital with access to a PC to search the library's

---

1. Stead EA, Jr. The National Library of Medicine: The great equalizer between small hospitals and major medical centers. *North Carolina Medical Journal*, 49:360, 1988.

immense Medline files. Medline, with some six million records, is a sort of online *Index Medicus*, but with abstracts.

The software itself is inexpensive. The cost of an average search, including all communication charges, is just $2 to $3. This is all it takes to have access to the latest published information on any medical topic. Your hospital librarian can even use NLM's Docline service to place an online order for a copy of an article!

In North Carolina only 34 of 160 hospitals have joined the National Library of Medicine's only network. By contrast 178 persons in our state—doctors, laboratories, businesses and students—have codes and are users of the world's most extensive store of medical information.

I suggest that each institution, regardless of size, place a terminal or PC where doctors congregate. If the Grateful Med software is used, the doctors should be encouraged to do their own searching. I would train a member of the hospital staff to assist the computerphobes. Thus, your staff will be on the same footing as the doctors at Duke, Carolina, East Carolina, Bowman Gray, and our other major medical centers.

Once my "computerized window" to the world of medical information was up and running, I'd turn to the public relations department and make sure the community knew about it. I'd have spots on local radio and television showing live patients and their doctors using up-to-date information to help with their care. I'd make it clear that patients would need to go to major medical centers only for major procedures; they would no longer need to go because their doctors were unsure of the latest medical information.

Finally, I'd let them know that their taxes paid for amassing this information, and that the few dollars spent on having access to it was money well spent for high-quality care.

Chapter 21

Computers, Doctors and Medical Students

C omputers are in widespread use in the life sciences.[1] More often than not computers in medical education and in the delivery of health care have been used by medical educators and physicians to improve the function of existing educational programs and health care delivery systems.[2] The Steering Committee believes that this approach is inadequate and that solutions for many of our problems will not be possible until we design new approaches. We will have to reexamine the problems in medical education and practice and devise solutions utilizing computer technology which will offer new approaches to education and give new patterns for professional staffing of clinical units, for the collection of clinical and laboratory data, and for clinical decision-making. We can no longer be bound indefinitely to the present mix of manpower that is produced by our educational institutions or by the present allocations of tasks to our current array of health professionals. These changes in medical education

1. Stead EA, Jr. Educational Technology for Medicine: Roles for the Lister Hill Center. Report of the Biomedical Communications Network Steering Committee Council of Academic Societies Association of American Medical Colleges, Part II, Chapter 6. Computers, supplement to *J. Med. Education* (now *Academic Medicine*), 59-66, 1971. Eugene Stead, Jr., was chairman of this committee.

2. National Academy of Sciences, Digital Computers in the Life Sciences. In *The Life Sciences*, Washington, DC: National Academy of Sciences, 1970.

and practice should be catalyzed by the Lister Hill Center. They cannot be realized without the development of strong research and educational programs in our major universities and medical centers. Mindful of the past and aware that the National Library of Medicine and its Lister Hill Center have never faced an educational program of this magnitude, we unhesitatingly recommend that the Lister Hill Center become the agency responsible for the development of the medical manpower for the computer science age in medical education and practice.

We must appreciate the differences in the reaction of medical educators and practicing physicians to multimedia audiovisual aids and to the use of computers in medical education and practice. The multimedia audiovisual aids are new and attractive forms of instruction which use the conventional words of the English language. The computer is different from these in that it demands a new language and has a capacity for the storage and retrieval of knowledge beyond that of any medium in which the physician has ever worked. It is likely to remain strange to most of the present practicing generation, and its use and acceptance will come only as the current generation of high school, college, and undergraduate medical students move into the various areas of medicine.

The Lister Hill Center and the National Library of Medicine are already involved in computer-oriented activities. Computerization is necessary to give the National Library of Medicine the ability to search the literature rapidly (MEDLARS), to keep the indices of medical publications and authors current, and to supply specialized bibliographies to researchers and clinicians. These functions are conducted in-house by staff of the National Library of Medicine and are financed as a part of its operational budget. The volume of work is large, the input of the data is under central control, and the printed output clearly serves the entire nation and world. The purpose of this chapter is to examine the future role of the computer scientist in biomedical education and in the development and dissemination of biomedical information.

The Steering Committee believes that the computer scientist will play an increasingly important role in medical education and practice. It envisions that eventually computer programs for obtaining quickly the best answer to a clinical problem, for the storage and retrieval of biologic data, for clinical simulation, for the maintenance of central medical records, for evaluation of educational programs, for clinical decision-making, and for medical curriculum planning will be written and made available for distribution through the Lister Hill Center.

The Lister Hill Center should develop the afferent and efferent arms of a communication network for computer scientists interested in biomedical education, research, delivery of personal health services, and construction of health care delivery systems. We still have to develop a useful and meaningful content which can be collated and processed by the Lister Hill Center for delivery to the efferent nodes which are to use the content. The Steering Committee believes that the concept of the network is important and that it will persist, regardless of changes in technology. The physical means by which the content flows from the periphery to the Lister Hill Center and back to the periphery will vary. For the present, we envisage the mail and the telephone as the important physical links. The Lister Hill Center should serve as a clearinghouse to coordinate the activities of other governmental agencies which are spending monies for hardware, for software, or for the development of programs in the broad field of health and biomedicine. The Lister Hill Center must have a staff that can establish criteria for the development of programs which will ensure their convertibility for distribution over a national network. It should be in a position to advise the universities and federal granting agencies about the ability of various combinations of hardware and software to meet the network requirements. The Lister Hill Center must establish criteria of excellence for content which will ensure that the material developed will have acceptability by a large number of the potential users.

The history of computer science suggests that rapid change and technological advancement are inherent. The advent of the large time-sharing computer is emerging simultaneously with that of the mini-computer. Which will be more technologically, educationally, and economically suitable for the applications in the health professions is undetermined at this point.

The Steering Committee believes that technological advancements concerning the characteristics of computer-oriented systems designed to facilitate economic and efficient information transfer should be carefully and continuously studied by or in the Lister Hill Center.

The Lister Hill Center can ensure that medical programs designed for computers dedicated to an area are developed in a way suitable for general use, that the developed programs are evaluated, and that the appropriate ones are selected for distribution by national and regional centers. Only time will determine the role of large, electronically connected time-share computers and the role of the small computers sharing programs which are sent by mail.

The question arises as to where the activities of the Lister Hill Center should stop. The Steering Committee takes the position that a large part of information useful for health planning, health operations, health care research, and education of health-related personnel will be programmed for computers and available for storage, retrieval, and distribution by the Lister Hill Center. The staff and facilities to accumulate, organize, and relay the data to the Lister Hill Center will have to be created throughout the nation. The function of the Lister Hill Center is to handle the central storage and retrieval mechanism as the data flow in from the periphery, to handle the distribution of the data throughout the nation, and to be an organizing and catalytic force to hasten the medical center and medical academia to do their share of the task. The following areas are ripe for development.

Manpower

Computer scientists and their tools are essential portions of modern managerial systems. The collection of data, their organization for storage and retrieval, the use of simulation in the manipulation of data, the setting-up of central record systems, the evaluation of the curriculum, and the collection and organization of data for community health planning are, in a broad way, managerial problems involving systems engineering and computer scientists. As yet, units creating computer scientists are not commonly available in most medical centers. When they are present, they are usually supported by research and service contracts and are rarely staffed by computer scientists knowledgeable about medicine or by physicians knowledgeable about computer science. University departments of computer science are usually located at a distance from the medical center, and few physicians, medical students, interns, or residents ever see them. Medical schools have had no way to finance departments of computer science, and the computer facilities in most medical centers have educated few computer scientists. Many persons examining the available hardware and software have envisaged major impacts of this technology on medical education and health care. The Steering Committee believes that these visions will come true eventually but not until the medical centers and universities perform their traditional job of producing manpower educated to function at the patient-doctor-manager interface. The National

Library of Medicine and the Lister Hill Center should make every effort to obtain money to fund initially approximately 10 regional medical computer science divisions in universities that have strong computer science programs. These units would have three functions:

1. To provide educational programs in the medical centers that offer advanced degrees to students from fields other than medicine who are interested in health sciences and which offer graduate education to medical students, interns, and residents who are interested in computer science.

2. To become involved in the development of computer programs for obtaining quickly the best answer to a clinical problem, for clinical simulation, for central medical records, for evaluation of educational programs, for clinical decision-making, for medical curriculum planning, and for health care system planning.

    These units should he the core facilities that feed material to the Lister Hill Center for correlation, storage, and distribution.

3. To develop standards for languages, hardware, and software to a degree sufficient to allow the free flow of material from one unit to another. The staffs of these units should meet at least four times a year with the permanent staff of the Lister Hill Center and the scholars-in residence at the Lister Hill Center.

The Steering Committee believes that in view of the size of the country, the number of persons who will have to be trained, the importance of the problems to be solved, and the necessity for the involvement of physicians at many levels, 10 centers represent the minimal investment which will be capable of initiating change.

Education of the Physician

Computer simulation has the potentiality of speeding up and enriching the present learning experiences of medical students as well as reducing the cost of teaching clinical medicine. In the past, the costs of converting a green team of medical students into a finished product capable of rendering complex professional services have been buried. The costs are of two types: (a) dollar costs for additional days in the hospital because it takes longer to carry out the diagnostic and therapeutic procedures with a green learning team than with a team of trained professionals; and (b) social costs because the longer time taken in giving the health care prolongs the length of time that the family undergoes a major disruption.

A reduction in the average stay of patients in hospitals with teaching responsibilities might be achieved by thoughtful and imaginative uses of the computer to simulate medical situations which might not otherwise be readily available to students. Situations have already been developed which offer the student the opportunity to manipulate data, make mistakes, get into trouble, and get out of trouble all without endangering patients using up valuable hospital time.

Dr. Stephen Abrahamson and associates at the University of Southern California have developed a simulation model known as Sim One to facilitate clinical training in anesthesia.[3] This life-

3. Abrahamson S, Denson JS, and Wolf RM. Effectiveness of a simulator in training anesthesiology residents. *J. Med. Educ.*, 44:515-519, 1969.

size mannequin has several functions, such as respiratory activity, pulse rate, blood pressure, skin color, and pupillary size which are under the computer's control. Each function responds to drug administration as well as to other interventions used by the anesthesiologist in managing patients in surgery. This model can be used by trainees to interact with a variety of situations that they will shortly encounter in real-life. They are allowed to deal with these situations repeatedly without risk to real patients and with immediate feedback about the effects of their judgments and actions.

Dr. William Harless and associates at the University of Illinois have developed a computer-aided simulation of the clinical encounter (CASE).[4] During the interactive session, the computer assumes the role of the patient, and the student assumes the role of the practicing physician. Virtually any type of patient with any variety of health problems can be simulated. A brief description of the patient and the setting appears on the terminal screen, after which the student begins the management process. Students use natural English language to direct questions to the "patient," request laboratory tests, or ask for physical information. They may obtain information from any of these resources at any time they choose. Ultimately, they must prescribe treatment to which the simulated patient responds. There are no unnatural cues, such as question sheets, to direct the path of inquiry students take and no artificial language required for their interaction with the simulated patient. The commitment to reality is the attribute that distinguishes CASE as an educational entity. Learning occurs from the students doing rather than from

---

4. Harless WG, Drennon GG, Marxer JJ, Root JA and Miller GE. CASE: A computer-aided simulation of the clinical encounter. *J. Med. Educ.*, 46:443–448, 1970.

their being told what to do. An extensive library of CASEs is being developed that will provide the student with the opportunity to interact with an unlimited number of simulated patients with various diseases while he is training to be a physician.

The experience of the air transportation industry suggests that this approach may be economically sound. Mechanical flight simulation equipment to train pilots was first used in World War II. This early equipment facilitated learning of coordinative motor skills to pilot an aircraft. Present-day simulators have kept pace with the increasing complexity of large jet aircraft and the resultant increasing demands on the air crew not only for skill but also for technical knowledge. Pilots now receive flight training in sophisticated aircraft simulators which are computer-controlled and programmed. Normal and abnormal flight conditions and changing situations are programmed into the simulated cockpit, the pilot's reactions are then fed into the program, and the computer predicts the flight results of his responses. A printout analysis is immediately available to student and instructor for corrections of errors and reinforcement of proper responses.

Although computers and associated simulation equipment are extremely costly, most major airlines have established multimillion-dollar educational facilities such as the United Airlines Flight Training Center in Denver. The airlines feel that simulation training is economical since the $10 per minute to run a simulated Boeing 747 compares favorably with the $80 per minute to maintain an airborne 747. They are able to train more people per week without problems of weather and schedule. Safety is another feature that impresses the airlines. Emergency flight conditions can be simulated which arc not safely possible in actual flights. Training accidents have been reduced. The efficiency of pilots in handling emergency situations is improved through experience, and the student and instructor have permanent computer records of emergency behavior which can be evaluated and compared with subsequent in training behavior.

Whenever possible, the Lister Hill Center should support the development and distribution of simulation programs which promise measurable educational gain. Due to the potential cost benefits, the Lister Hill Center should encourage exploration of these programs by the Social Security Administration and other agencies responsible for paying for medical care.

The Lister Hill Center should also demonstrate how medical units in a given city might work together and eventually develop programs for two cities working together. The peripheral units must be developed before there is any strength in networking.

Accumulation of Data for Answering Clinical Questions

As the staff supported by computer scientists work for the best answer to a clinical problem, they will find that the data needed to make this judgment frequently are not available. With the computer doing the memory work, each diagnostic category can he profitably broken down into many more subgroups than we have been able to describe in conventional textbooks. The records of patients as presently kept cannot supply the needed data because the physicians collecting the data have used them for immediate purposes and were not concerned with creating data to be used for text book purposes. The National Library of Medicine will have to face up eventually to the reality of the situation. Accurate data can be collected, but they have to be collected for the specific purpose of establishing appropriate subgroups. The expense of collecting the data can be borne in part by the patient, but a considerable amount of the expense must be charged to the expense of developing a computerized library.

New persons must be developed at the physician-patient-computer interface to collect, verify, and feed the data into the system. The Lister Hill Center and the National Library of Medicine can develop the capability for analyzing the data and making them available throughout the nation. The more difficult task is to mobilize the 50 to 100 medical centers, each of which would be responsible for continuous input of data covering the areas for which they have accepted responsibility.

The Lister Hill Center must work with professional organizations to begin to assemble the pieces which can then be assembled into larger units. The Myocardial Infarction Research Units of the National Heart and Lung Institute[1] could write the definitive work on the natural history of myocardial infarction. These 10 regional units could form an input network to the Lister Hill Center for national distribution. Committees of the national health societies or of the professorial associations now active in every discipline are resources that could be tapped.

It is easy to measure the amount of material that a candidate has memorized. It is difficult to test the ability of the candidate to use the material in a variety of situations. Computer simulation offers a new approach to this problem. As mentioned earlier in this chapter, some systems already exist where the data from virtually any patient can be programmed and used as a simulation for purposes of instruction or examination. The Lister Hill Center should explore, with the National Board of Medical Examiners and the Advisory Boards for Medical Specialties, their activities in these areas and work with them wherever possible.

------

1. See Chapter 46, This Volume, "The Opportunities for a Research Professor on Myocardial Infarction: The Report of the NIH Ad Hoc Committee," p. 327-358.

Health Care Delivery—Making Available to the Physician the Best Answer to Any Clinical Question

This will involve the National Library of Medicine and its Lister Hill Center in a new function, and it will require the development of new relationships with the academic community. When the National Library of Medicine does a bibliography search, it does not weigh the value of the articles listed, and it cannot produce a weighing of the material without a working cadre of physicians. The National Library of Medicine will need space and budget to support the staff updating this yesterday's "best available answer." Much of the compilation and revision should be done by persons working in the Lister Hill Center during leave of absence from universities, varying from three to 18 months. These persons could be called scholars-in-residence.

Computer-Aided Decision-Making

At present, there are conventional ways of introducing patients into the medical care system, of collecting data, and of making decisions about diagnosis, prognosis, and treatment. The present attempts to introduce computers into medical centers are about improving these conventional ways. We try to make the present better. More likely, the major impact from computer scientists and their hardware will come when the old systems are discarded and new ones developed. We may well discover that the physician can have a larger role as a manager, that technicians can make primary observations now made by physicians, and that computers can calculate strategies and possibilities better than can the physician.[5] Computer-aided diagnosis with no

---

5. Schwartz WB. Medicine and the computer: The promise and problems of change. *New Eng. J. Med.*, 283:1257-1264, 1970.

commitment to following the usual thinking of the physician should be tried in at least five specialty areas.

Some 40 million people in rural areas might gain access to basic medical care through exploration of new technology. If this were possible, expenditures of large magnitude would be justified, particularly if practical alternatives either were not available or were more expensive.

The Lister Hill Center should work cooperatively with the National Center for Health Services Research and Development of the Health Services and Mental Health Administration in the development of programs for clinical decision-making.

Health Care Planning

Medical centers, hospitals, medical schools, and regional health areas all have a number of identifiable subsystems that must be interrelated, budgeted, and operated. Data must be collected to characterize the subsystems as they now exist and to examine the advantages and disadvantages of possible alternatives. What will be the effect of enlarging the student body on the requirements for teaching beds? Can these be met in one hospital with the addition of a summer quarter, or will an additional clinical affiliation be required? How many ambulatory patients need to he cared for to fill a given number of inpatient beds? How does this decision affect the need of the X-ray department for space? How many beds need to be built in what areas of the country? Which services should be kept in all hospitals and which should be eliminated from some and concentrated in others?

In time, the medical history will begin with birth and the examination of the infant. It will be updated in grammar school, high school, and college. It will need to be storable and to be retrievable. Again, the Lister Hill Center cannot impose this change on the country, but it can be the catalyst that starts the planning and the pilot operations. The U.S. Office of Education and the child health program could be encouraged to conduct pilot programs.

Chapter 22

Biomedical Instructional Technology: The State of the Art

The Medium Is Not the Message

Instructional technology has been regarded as the new media, born of the 20th century communications and electronics revolution and designed to supplement or replace teacher, textbook, and blackboard.[1] Unfortunately this attitude has led to a hardware- and system-orientation which pays little attention to the message and its role in the learning process.

A more recent educational attitude goes beyond any medium or machine and regards instructional technology as "a systematic way of designing, carrying out, and evaluating the total process of learning and teaching in terms of the specific objectives, based on research in human learning and communication, and employing a combination of human and non-human resources to bring about more effective instruction" Multimedia technology in American education is low both in quantity and quality. The use of films, film strips, records, programmed texts, television, and computer programs accounts for one to five percent of learning time for 50 million students in the United States.

---

1. Stead, E.A., Jr. Educational Technology for Medicine: Roles for the Lister Hill Center. Report of the Biomedical Communications Network Steering Committee Council of Academic Societies Association of American Medical Colleges, Part II, Chapter 2. supplement to *J. Med. Education* (now *Academic Medicine*), 21-28, 1971. Eugene Stead, Jr. was chairman of this committee.

In 1969, $1.4 billion were spent for audiovisual products, personnel, and their services. At the present rate of expansion in this industry, annual expenditures up to $4.0 billion are predicted by 1980. While the American public was spending $625 million for software (film, slides, audiotape, and videotape), they purchased equipment worth $427 million.[2]

It is interesting to note that all segments of the market, including public schools and colleges, spent from 5 to 15 percent more, except medicine and public health. These areas showed a five percent decline in purchases[3] compared with a 20 percent increase in 1968.[4] In view of inflationary trends, these data reflect increased or stable audiovisual sales and services for education in general while suggesting a decline in use by the health sciences. Decreased federal funds for training programs and research may account for this.

A 1969 National Conference on the Use of Audiovisuals in Medical Education[5] summarized the present-day multimedia technology and its usefulness and limitations in biomedical education. Apart from economic factors, it is obvious from this report that the major limitations in instructional technology are not due to the quality or variety of available hardware, software format, or the ability to create interacting systems. The quality of the content (the message) and its presentation, the choice of

---

2. Commission on Instructional Technology. To Improve Learning: A Report to the President and the Congress of the United States by the Commission on Instructional Technology. Washington, DC: United States Government Printing Office, 1970.

3. A.V. Buying in 1969. ETV Newsletter #96, July 27, 1970.

4. Market Review: Non-theatrical film and audiovisual, 1968. *J. Society Motion Pictures and T.V. Engineers*, 78:973-988, 1969.

5. The Proceedings of a National Conference on the Use of Audiovisual in Medical Education at the University of Alabama Medical Center, August 6-8, 1969.

the proper media (audio, film, T.V., slide, sound, etc.), and the ability to meet the needed educational objectives are more important limiting factors.

The 1970 Presidential and Congressional Report on Instructional Technology amplifies this limitation in general education while stressing the widespread ineffectiveness of a media-oriented approach especially where a single medium is stressed.

Instructional Technology and the Teacher

Teachers in medical schools may be knowledgeable in their fields of science and clinical practice, but their ability to transfer knowledge, enthusiasm, and the desire to learn to students varies from poor to superb. Attempts to teach medical teachers how to teach and how to evaluate their own effectiveness are as yet miniscule compared with the need.[6] Research in medical education is still deficient.[7] Selection of medical school faculty members has been more often based on interest in research rather than on teaching skill. This scene appears to be changing, however, both in the developing medical schools and in some of those that are well-established. Resistance to instructional technology is decreased. Biomedical teachers are becoming more alert to new pedagogy needed to accompany curricular reforms. The decrease in research funds has shifted faculty attention toward teaching and health care delivery. Now a young academician may be encouraged and perhaps rewarded for developing teaching interests and skills in the various instructional technologies.

Training programs to prepare medical educators in the principles of learning, teaching, and evaluation now exist in at least

6. Fleisher DS. Medical education: A clinical pathologic conference. *Med. Clin. N. Amer.*, 54:591-602, 1970.

7. Sanazaro PJ. The information gap in medical education. *J. Med. Educ.*, 40:221-222, 1965.

four medical centers. These centers are instrumental in providing educational specialists for other health science schools. Programs to develop instructional skills and manpower in the audiovisual and computer technologies are less conspicuous and are not well advertised. Training programs, however, which integrate the learning and educational aspects with media training are being encouraged and should be available in increased numbers in the near future.

Audiovisual specialists, biomedical teachers, and educational specialists are beginning to relate to each other through conferences. In individual medical school faculties, these groups join to evaluate educational needs as a basis for providing supplemental materials in the proper media and to evaluate the materials and their influence on the student's professional behavior.

Such an Approach Is Still the Exception Rather than the Rule

The average biomedical teacher does not have funds, time, or necessary technical assistance at his disposal to produce supplemental multimedia materials; so he must borrow or do without. He is frequently unable to locate adequate audiovisual materials produced by others in specific content areas he needs. If he can identify the existence of audiovisual materials, he is usually unable to obtain them without months of prior notice, which is frequently impossible in the clinical and elective programs. This serves as a deterrent to the instructor to search and seek supplemental materials.

The lack of a central index and catalog of multimedia materials and the absence of a sharing system for multimedia materials are limitations that hamper the faculty at all medical schools but which most seriously affect those whose schools have the most limited budgets.

For this study, site visits were made to medical schools, and consultations were conducted with selected faculty in other settings as well. From these interviews, a number of attitudes emerged. For some faculty, externally generated teaching aids threaten the self-image of their scientific and instructional authority. Specifically cited fears were loss of status, job replacement, competitive informational and curriculum control, and dehumanization. Fears of governmental control, loss of objectivity if supported by pharmaceutical companies, and an antipathy toward slick media professionalism were all reported to inhibit acceptance and exchange of audiovisual materials between schools and with federal and industrial lenders.

In general, the faculties of dentistry and nursing schools accept and use audiovisual supplemental materials more than do schools of medicine. The basic science faculties which are more accustomed to presenting didactic lectures to large classes accept educational technology more readily and produce more audiovisual materials than do the clinical faculties which work with smaller groups teaching clinical skills in the tutorial tradition. Open rejection has been converted to acceptance when the educational technology was demonstrated to increase the efficiency of the teacher, especially if he must repeat the same message many times each year to small groups.

Teachers presenting lectures or seminars in areas peripheral to their own specialty interests are more prone to accept externally generated content and to use supplemental audiovisual materials. This is an increasingly important factor since few, if any, schools or departments can afford a complete faculty covering all specialty and subspecialty areas and the increasingly important interdisciplinary correlations.

A biomedical teacher is still responsible for his own curriculum and the content being delivered whether by himself or by an audiovisual presentation that he has chosen. The media, by virtue of user response, will probably always be secondary to the message in medical education, but there are content areas with naturally lend themselves to various media. When a media to message compatibility is obvious to the teacher, he is more interested in producing or using supplemental materials. For example, many neurologists are interested in producing or using films or T.V. tapes that display the neurological examination and disturbances of movement and behavior. Surgeons utilize motion media to show and evaluate operative skills. Heart sounds go on audiotapes and oscilloscopes, which are naturally recorded by cardiologists.

Strident enthusiasm and motivation to learn and to perform well, however, still come from a smile, a word, and a push. This very important contribution from the live teacher is not as yet simulated by other media. Furthermore, man — not materials, nor systems, nor institutions — must again be the focus of education and the focus of human concern before the conflicts and frustrations of all higher education can be resolved.[8] It is the teacher's responsibility to maintain this orientation.

Instructional Technology and the Student

Student Attitudes

Today's medical students are different. They are openly more aggressive and critical of teachers and teaching. They demand curricular relevance and a voice in curricular and administrative decisions. They maintain that they are better educated, better informed, and more concerned about medical practice in their community than were their predecessors. They have yet to

---

8. Chickering A. Preface in *Education and Identity*, Jossey-Bass, 1969.

demonstrate evidence of any increased responsibility or more dedicated behavior than earlier generations of students.

Today's medical students have grown with television as a babysitter; so they accept the media. They will passively watch a bad movie, but they refuse to become intellectually involved with poorly presented or seemingly unimportant biomedical materials; so they avoid medical T.V. presentations unrelated to their curricula, patients, or examinations. They respond adversely to multimedia materials much as they would to a personal presentation which they consider irrelevant, of poor quality, or pitched either beneath or over their heads. Once these objections are met, today's students enthusiastically accept communications technology if, in addition, interested faculty are available and functioning aggressively to supplement or complement their technologically-based learning experiences or to demand evidence of their having learned the media-presented message.

Self-Instruction

Individualized instruction and the mechanisms and materials to facilitate it are more necessary in today's climate of student and curricular heterogeneity. Properly done, it demands a more active student involvement than passive classroom behavior. Self-instruction is more important to the school and faculty because, though new curricula and larger student numbers have not brought more faculty, they are bringing more elective courses, smaller student groups, and wider geographic dispersal. Self-instructional, media-oriented programs are, therefore, increasing each year in the medical sciences. One noteworthy example is the neurosciences study program at the University of California, San Diego, whose tutorial environment offers audiovisuals, models, programmed instruction guides, and printed material for neurosciences self-instruction.

A well-defined core curriculum lends itself to the development of self-instructional media systems. Many departments of obstetrics and gynecology have defined such a core curriculum. By sharing with each other, they have produced self-instructional environments with a core content composed of books, programmed texts, audiotapes, and audiovisual cartridges utilized by the small groups of students who appear on their OB-GYN service every six weeks. After students complete the media "core," the faculty then present more sophisticated material in their clinical interactions with the students.

Audiovisual Media

Motion pictures and television for large classes have been used in biomedical education for several decades. The popularity of small group and individual audiovisual usage is recent. Self-contained software cartridges or cassettes and small rear view projectors bring instant replays where motion is needed, but their hardware and software lack standardization and fool-proof construction.

Television in biomedical education has found new applications in perfecting the interviewing and examining skills of students. A replay of interview and examination of the patient is made, and the instructor and student can evaluate at their leisure the quality of the student's performance.

Video playback systems which allow for small, self-contained software units to be played through home T.V. were recently demonstrated and have been promised for delivery in 1971. This innovation may well revolutionize the individual teacher's and student's ability to produce and duplicate inexpensively self-instructional audiovisual materials for individual and small group usage.

Computer-Assisted — Biomedical Instruction

The past five years have seen the development of several different types of computer-assisted instructional approaches in biomedical education.[9,10] Several schools are offering electives in computer applications in medicine and education.[11] The use of computers in medical education is clearly rising.[12]

Basically, the computer can be used as a tool to drill the student in rote memory of medical knowledge, which is far more expensive than a book or a chart, or it can in some ways present cues and programmed responses to guide the student's decision-making process, judgments, and organizational skills. The computer and its programs can act to collect data, simulate a patient, simulate a tutor, or simulate a physician.

The Computer as a Data Collector. Slack[13] has devised a patient interviewing program. The computer interrogates the patient to gather his medical record. This type program allows for patient education, as well as providing an information bank for student learning, patient care, or research retrieval. The physical examination is also recorded by the computer rather than dictated or written by the physician.[14]

---

9. Stolourow LM, Peterson II, and Cunningham AC. *Computerized-assisted Instruction in the Health Profession.* Newburyport, MA: ENTELEK 1970.

10. Harless WG. Computer assisted medical education. In *Handbook of Biomedical Information Systems.* Encyclopedia Britannica. in press.

11. Yoder RD. A course in biomedical computing applications. *J. Med. Educ.*, 44:1056-1062, 1969.

12. Hubbard WN, Gronvall JA, and Demuth GR. The medical school curriculum. *J. Med. Educ.*, 45:November, Part 2, 1970.

13. Slack W., Hicks CP, Reed, CE, and Vancura LJ. A computer-based medical-history system. *New Eng. J. Med.*, 274:194-198, 1966.

14. Slack WV, Peckham BM, Vancura LJ, and Carr WFA. A computer-based physical examination system. *JAMA*, 200:224-228, 1967.

A problem-oriented medical record[15] devised by Weed differs in that the student is systematically guided to enter the information he gathered from the patient's history and physical examination into the computer to arrive logically at a diagnosis and to remain orderly and logical as he cares for the patient in a problem-oriented fashion. This program has the virtue of being a guidance system which can be used without a computer.

The Computer as a Teacher. Early programs at the University of Oklahoma offered tutorial queries in a Socratic dialogue in anatomy, medicine, physiology, and anesthesiology.[16,17,18] Other schools have developed programs in pathology, nuclear medicine, and clinical diagnosis, to name only a few.[19,20,21]

Computer-based tutorial programs in all basic sciences are now being used at Ohio State. These programs arc also capable of evaluating the effectiveness of the computer's information

---

15. Weed LL. *Medical Records, Medical Education and Patient Care.* Cleveland, Ohio: Case Western Reserve Press, 1969.

16. Proceedings, Conference on the Use of Computers in Medical Education at the University of Oklahoma Medical Center, April 3-5,1968. Co-sponsored by U.S. Department of H.E.W., Public Health Service, Bureau of Health Manpower, and University of Oklahoma School of Medicine, April 3-5, 1968.

17. Harless WG, Lucas NC, Cutter A, Duncan RC, White JM, and Brandt E. Computer-assisted instruction in continuing medical education. *J. Med. Educ.*, 44:670-674, 1969.

18. Thies R, Harless WC, Lucas NC, and Jacobson FD. An experiment comparing computer-assisted instruction with lecture presentation in physiology. *J. Med. Educ.*, 44:1156-1160, 1969.

19. Bowden DH. Computer-aided instruction in pathology. *Canad. Med. Ass. J.*, 97:739-742, 1967.

20. Brown DW, Groome DS, Nichoff RD, and Cleaveland JD. Computer-assisted instruction in nuclear medicine. *JAMA*, 206:1059-1062, 1968.

21. Dombal FT, de Hartley JR, and Steeman DH. A computer-assisted system for learning clinical diagnosis. *Lancet*, 1:145-148, 1969.

transfer by utilizing the computer s ability to catalog the student's progress. In this environment, students are immersed in computer guidance, and the early evaluations sound guardedly enthusiastic. Many other programs exist but are unknown outside their own schools.

The Computer as a Patient. This type of instructional program has been developed to the present capability by Harless[22] and Barnett.[23] Barnett's uses a limited interacting language to test the effectiveness of the student's clinical decisions by the step-wise management of the simulated patient. Evaluation mechanisms are also built into these systems. The Sim One patient simulator for anesthesiology training is a noteworthy example.

Patient simulation programs now appear to offer more potential for assisting the developing of clinical judgment than other types of educational media experiences available to an expanding body of students.

The Computer as a Physician. Several plans and programs for clinical consultation and decision-making by the computer exist. The best examples are in electrolyte and fluid balance management[24,25] and EKG interpretation.[26] Some of these programs have educational value, but most are basically labor-saving devices.

22. Harless WG. Computer-assisted medical education. In *The Computer Utility: Implications for Higher Education.* Lexington, MA: D.C. Heath and Company, 1970.

23. Gorry CA, and Barnett GO. Experience with a model of sequential diagnosis. *Computers and Biomedical Research,* 1:49-507, 1968.

24. Schwartz WB. Medicine and the computer: The promise and problems of change. *New Eng. J. Med.,* 283:1257-1264, 1970.

25. Bleich HL. The computer as a consultant. *New Eng. J. Med.,* 284:141-147, 1971.

26. Caceres CA, and Hochbero HM. Performance of the computer and physician in the analysis of the electrocardiogram. *Amer. Heart J.,* 79:439-443, 1970.

Postgraduate and Continuing Education

Residency training programs are finding some value in the use of television and motion pictures for modifying diagnostic and manual skills of housestaff as well as students.[27] Self-assessment programs for practitioners are being placed on a computer format by the University of Washington's Regional Medical Program.

Telephone dial-access programs giving a wide variety of five-minute lectures on many medical topics are available through the continuing education efforts of both the University of Wisconsin and the University of Missouri. The University of Alabama offers telephone consultation services to practitioners on patient-related problems.

When they become available, video playback materials will have the best promise of providing educational packages for both information transfer and self-assessment to the practicing physician that he can observe in his own living room on his own T.V.

The monthly audio cassette programs now available afford the busy physician an opportunity to listen to material while driving a car.

The Lister Hill Center's new experiment of putting the *Abridged Index Medicus* in an on-line computer base for retrieval by a phone coupled terminal offers students, faculty, house staff, and practitioners a bibliographic service from which they can request hard copy from their nearby medical library, regional medical library, or regional medical program.

Probably the most effective method of medical self-renewal today for the individual physician is found in those medical

---

27. Peltier LF, Geertsma RH, and Youmans RL. Television videotape recording: An adjunct in teaching emergency medical care. *Surgery*, 66:233–236, 1969.

schools which provide practitioners with an opportunity to return to the medical center for several weeks of uninterrupted study and active participation with faculty and housestaff in day to day patient care and learning sessions. The physician participating in such a program also has ready access to all library and audiovisual materials. At least 14 specialty societies are now offering or are planning to sponsor self-assessment programs: American Academy of Obstetrics and Gynecology, American Academy of Orthopaedic Surgeons, American Academy of Ophthalmology and Otolaryngology, American Academy of Pediatrics, American Association of Neurological Surgeons, American College of Cardiology, American College of Physicians, American College of Radiology, American College of Surgeons, American Council of Otolaryngology, American Psychiatric Association, American Society of Clinical Pathologists, American Society of Plastic and Reconstructive Surgeons, and College of American Pathologists. These programs should stimulate physicians' self-educational activities and should also increase the need for a biomedical communications network and local and regional continuing education programs. It goes without saying that if recertification and relicensure laws are enacted, the demand for self-assessment and self-instructional programs will explode.

Undergraduate Medical Education

A 1968 survey of curricular development in United States and Canadian medical schools suggests that new curricular changes may be responsible for a two- to three-fold increase in the use of audiovisual and computer materials, programmed instruction, and simulation techniques. This implies that both faculty and administration of most schools are increasing their interest in and support for instructional technology.

The learning resource units that receive the most faculty support and provide the most service are those which also have allocated funds to produce content for venturing teachers. Most such units around the country have concentrated their efforts on local production and have not provided comprehensive search and delivery service for materials produced elsewhere.

Some audiovisual production units produce extremely sophisticated materials at high cost. If used only locally, they are hardly worth their price. Other audiovisual departments provide internal networks of classroom and laboratory television service from a central studio. Their educational value and utilization increase with their ability to use external materials as well.

Although most schools either now have or are planning audiovisual and or instructional technology divisions, these units are frequently understaffed and poorly funded. In spite of these constraints, they are still able to serve as a local nidus on which the Lister Hill Center could provide supporting service to faculty and students. These constraints are a reason for the existence of a biomedical communications network.

Audiovisual and computer materials are expensive to write and produce. An inordinate number of faculty hours go into their production. These costs can be reclaimed by widespread use of the materials. A faculty member wishing so to invest his time must search for support, usually outside his own school. The time consumed in locating and obtaining financial support and in design and production is an inevitable expense which is far more significant to the teacher than costs of tape, technological equipment, and technical assistance. When these not inconsiderable costs of time and money are added together, sharing the produced materials through a network is not only realistic but also mandatory for efficient educational planning in the health science schools of tomorrow.

Today's Technology and Tomorrow's Lister Hill Center

Biomedical educational and its supporting audiovisual communications are the victims of a non-standardized industry which offers its buyers non-standardized hardware and software, incompatible from company to company and occasionally even between successive models from the same maker. The educator who plans to borrow audiovisual materials will find that his 8mm cartridge projector or videotape player is probably riot compatible with the borrowed or rented software. He must either pay more money to convert the materials to his format or buy other hardware. The video recorder and its software format are the least standardized. The newer video playback systems with widely different software format promise to be even more frustrating. Some hope, however, may be found in the Japanese industries' attempts to standardize video playback systems.

The problems of standardization, compatibility, and convertibility in computers and their software create even more complex problems that are not easily resolved when attempting to convert a computer-assisted instructional program to a system other than that on which it was designed.

Realizing the significance of this problem, the Lister Hill Center requested that the National Bureau of Standards undertake a study of the problems of standardization and convertibility inherent in planning a biomedical communications network.[28] This study is lengthy and complex, but in summary it recognizes that: (1) Standardization activities should make information

---

28. Stevens ME. Standardization, Compatibility and/or Convertibility Requirements in Network Planning. National Bureau of Standards Report 10-252. Washington, DC: United States Government Printing Office, 1970.

transferable rather than make it identical; (2) The problems are formidable and need instant attention, but they are not insurmountable in view (of the recent success of the three national libraries: the National Agricultural Library, the Library of Congress, and the National Library of Medicine, in adopting a standardized format for transmission of bibliographic information on magnetic tape; and (3) The Lister Hill Center is operating in an unprecedented field of network planning and should seize the leadership for standardization.

Networks

A number of medical schools in the past five years have presented one-way television programs to their medical community over the educational channels. The physicians' response to these programs has been as disappointing to the originators as the general quality of the content was to those who occasionally viewed them.

Interacting networks using single media have been used sparsely in medical education for over 20 years, first by phone and wireless and next by one-way television. In 1965, the first two-way video system was established in a medical school.[29]

Other interacting networks now exist for education and clinical consultation, and more are contemplated.

The problems of acceptance and rejection are similar to other media efforts. The network is successful only when it transmits something both needed and wanted in an acceptable fashion. Television networks per se are best received and most efficiently utilized where the participants and educators are the instigators, program planners, and content evaluators. When

---

29. Titus GW. Kansas University Medical Center Television: Two Decades, 1949-1969. *J. Kansas Med. Soc.*, 71:73-75, 1970.

content is poor and not related to the ongoing curriculum, the programs play to empty chairs.

Computer-assisted instructional programs have been shared recently among several hospitals through a commercial time-sharing corporation. Using phone coupled terminals, this type of network can be extended across the country. The line charges and time-sharing costs, however, make this quite expensive. Current problems with overloaded circuits and inordinate numbers of line changes add a series of technical barriers to the economic constraints which may be overcome by regional time sharing nodes in the network. The existing network, through the Regional Medical Library System, utilizes regional nodes for bibliographic search and retrieval service to schools and individuals. This system can be valuable to other biomedical communication services.

Chapter 23

Computerized Medical Practice: Old Dreams and Current Realties

C omputers have a certain fascination for those who have spent their careers developing young minds to explore unchartered waters.[1,2] Exposed naked to the world, men and women have too little force to make a major impact on their environment; but armed with instruments of their own creation, they have tremendous power to perturbate and even destroy large parts of the world.

With the development of speech, writing, and printing, information could be saved and transferred. Mankind could start with stored information and ascend to new plateaus. But books, charts, and journals were passive aids. Each brain had to assimilate and process available information before it could advance the store of knowledge. Now, computers allow information to be stored and manipulated in ways previously restricted to the brain. For the first time, humans are extending not only the power of arms and legs, but also brainpower.

---

1. Stead EA, Jr. and Stead WW. Computers and medical practice: Old dreams and current realities. *MD Computing*, 2:26–31, 1985.

2. This essay was co-authored by Dr. Stead's son, William W. (Bill) Stead, now Professor of Medicine and Computer Science and Vice-Chancellor of Vanderbilt University. Bill Stead is the architect of the Vanderbilt Medical Center medical information system.

DNA from egg and sperm dictates the structure of the brain; but after the first cell division, feedback from the environment becomes important. The result is a biological machine, which is programmed to carry out many functions before the infant leaves the womb. The combination of continued DNA programming and environmental factors leads to the adult brain.

The computer is a tool created and programmed by people. We all agree that there are no computers on the horizon with the flexibility and reprogramming ability of the brain. The combination of multiple sensory inputs, rich association pathways, and many motor outlets give the brain a large lead. Early dreams of using computers to review lifetime medical records and apply the wisdom of several specialists to an individual patient's care remain unfulfilled.

The future is less certain. In the last fifty years, computers have repeatedly increased their range of function. The brain has developed over millions of years; it is doubtful that significant biological improvements will occur in the next thousand. Major mutations increasing the power of the brain occur slowly, one at a time, so diffusion through the world's population is very slow. On the other hand, millions of individuals can join in constructing computers. Over time, they may develop a nonbiological system as complex and functional as the human brain, making our dreams come true.

The Evolution of Computers in Medicine: Successes and Failures

Twenty years ago, the National Institutes of Health and the National Aeronautics and Space Administration recognized that introducing computers into bioscience laboratories might open up many new areas of investigation. Computers at that time were large, bulky instruments guarded by computer scientists, programmers, and technicians. They were housed in specially air-conditioned buildings, far from working bioscience laboratories. They were too remote to be integrated into day-to-day research. A way was needed to unleash the creativity of the biomedical researcher.

The way turned out to be a standardized laboratory computer, small enough to be a working laboratory instrument, and easy for non-computer-trained researchers to program. Fred Stone, director of the Institute of General Medical Sciences, and Bruce Waxman, executive secretary of the Computer Science Study Section, arranged for financing. The Institute of General Medical Sciences supplied $3,200,000; the Institute of Mental Health $300,000; and NASA transferred $600,000 to General Medical Sciences for the venture. Wesley Clark, Willliam Papian, Charles Molnar, and others of the M.I.T. faculty created the LINCs computer. Scientists were able to acquire one of the 16 LINCs by submitting a research protocol and agreeing to spend two months at M.I.T., learning to assemble and service a computer to be located in the laboratory. When the bioscientists left the workshop with their new tool, the minicomputer and personal-computer era was on its way. Computers had been placed directly in the hands of scientists and this produced many creative new uses for the technology.

Medical Literature

The National Library of Medicine recognized that information was exploding and that old methods of cataloging sources or searching scientific literature were no longer adequate. They created Medline sparked by Martin Cummings. This computerized system supplied a complete set of references for any medical topic. Today the system is very sophisticated; you can specify subgroups much more definitely, and eliminate most of the irrelevant titles. The group at Beth Israel Hospital in Boston have made their library more user-friendly through a program called Paper Chase.

The terminals in a modern medical library are in constant use. The librarian's ability to identify sources of interest from only a modicum of input is constantly amazing. We no longer need to focus our efforts on finding facts; we can spend our time synthesizing them.

Practice Management

In the clinical areas, physicians' great expectations were not realized. Instead, computers entered large clinics and hospitals as tools of the accounting office. Even here, change was slow because the computer was only used to speed up standard accounting methods. For example, accountants used the computer to generate a batch report that would identify records missing a diagnosis, rather than using it interactively to prevent the creation of a record without specifying a diagnosis.

New approaches based on the capabilities of the new tools appeared slowly. With on-line computing, orders can be entered and a charge made when each order is filled, eliminating the need for an audit trail. Much of the paperwork can be eliminated, but on-line accountants love paper and are slow to change.

Accounting personnel had no incentive to experiment with clinical uses of computers. In those areas where doctors have developed medical information systems, there has been little crosstalk between the business office and the clinic. One group rarely knows what hardware and software are in other parts of the institution, and future purchases are often planned by one group without regard for other users. Thus, the users have not achieved cost savings by eliminating redundant special purpose hardware such as graphics or laser printers, neither have they increased their systems' reliability through shared backup facilities nor increased the functionality through networking.

Education and Clinical Assistance

In the last thirty years a number of eager beavers have created a large variety of databases for teaching, for assisting with patient care, and for guiding diagnosis. Most of these are rarely used. Medical schools do not yet recognize computer science as an important component of the curriculum. Medical schools and hospitals do not support computerized information systems in their budgets. Database creators have largely been entrepreneurs supported by non-institutional funds. Operating outside the traditional medical practice, they have usually failed to engage doctors in using their systems routinely. When the entrepreneur leaves, the computer program disappears.

Attitudes and Other Obstacles

One recurring problem has been the seduction of some doctors by computers. As a result, few persons writing medical information systems have continued to practice medicine. They have created a great variety of interesting material that is useless in practice. The average physician overestimates the accuracy and the usefulness of written information in traditional medical charts. When asked what information should be stored in the computer, the reply is "I need everything." When that advice is followed, the computer record becomes as overloaded and unworkable as its manual counterpart. We need teams of practicing doctors who are knowledgeable about software, and engineers who are comfortable as colleagues.

Most doctors have been slow to lay hands on the computer. They have not entered information directly into the system or extracted needed data from the computer themselves. Because they have employed interface personnel for these functions, a system has had to bear this overhead. However, the overhead for this isolation is greater than just the salaries. The support personnel ask the computer to do what they think the doctor wants. Since the doctor frequently does not understand the computer's capabilities and the support personnel do not understand the doctor's needs, the effort is wasted.

Computer software for practice has usually had narrowly focused purposes such as billing, checking for interactions between drugs, interpreting electrocardiograms, calculating values for pulmonary function testing, or interpreting blood gas and electrolyte data in renal failure. Most of the practice continues without using the computer. For this reason, the doctor is not involved in developing a new mode for his practice, and the computer is under-used. For example, while the computer prints prescriptions, it could be silently checking for drug-drug interactions. This type of cross-talk is rarely built into the system, because the doctor is peripheral to the venture.

Physicians think of computerization when facing an administrative problem such as processing insurance forms on time or rescheduling a day's appointments. Each practice's day-to-day routine is a patchwork of procedures evolved to solve past problems. Unless the computer is mentioned, the first thought is to use it to speed existing processes; this instinct overlooks the fact that taking full advantage of a computer requires that old processes be replaced. One way to schedule appointments is to divide the day into units, each of which is the size of the shortest appointment, and to let the secretary flip the pages of a book until she sees the right number of units for each patient. Such a system is flexible but depends on human visual ability to level the workload. The physician may have one day with six new patients, followed by a day with forty returns. Using a computer to keep a book that is visually managed is more tedious than using a paper book. If a physician accepts the discipline imposed by the computer and gives up the flexibility of personally establishing time schedules of different types and lengths, the computer can be used to match patients to resources, resulting in a more efficient practice.

Customizing a program to fit a physician's habits is expensive in time. In today's programs, sophisticated data dictionaries allow nonprogrammers to tailor a system to their needs; but developing and maintaining the dictionaries can require months of the doctor's time. Each procedure performed by a practice must be defined. Coding data requires listing all the items usually scribbled under "others" in a paper system. Defining the systems and then encoding the data is hard work; but once you have it in the computer, you can arrange the data in many ways and get a variety of useful outputs.

The doctor is a better diagnostician than the computer. Initially, all diagnoses are possible for a patient. The doctor quickly narrows the range until only a few possibilities remain. In many areas, the computer could be used at this stage to determine the most likely diagnosis. However, that doctor generally faces one of two situations. Either the doctor is an expert in evaluating the data because the practice has many patients with similar sets of problems—in which case computer evaluation is unnecessary—or else the doctor sees very few patients with the given set of problems—in which case no computer program is readily available to cover the issues at hand; it is much simpler to refer the patient to the appropriate specialist.

Interacting with a computer consultation program is not as rewarding as consulting with a specialist. Primary physicians can consult another physician for exactly what they want to know, slipping over known and understood facts. A computer program straightforward enough to be used by a novice is likely to force a more experienced user through a tedious dialogue. The specialist provides a dual function of caring for the patient and educating the primary physician. The primary physician in turn educates the specialist by providing follow-up data about the patient. Although the computer program may educate the physician, it normally learns nothing from the interchange.

Diagnostic programs go out of date rapidly. Since no one is really using them, their format is rigid and not easily modified. Because they are not widely used, no one knows how many modifications would be needed to help all the doctors who did not have a hand in writing the given program. There are no ready made methods to keep programs up-to-date and user-friendly. Artificial-intelligence techniques attempt to solve this problem by placing medical information in a database that can be changed by non-programming physicians, but the experimental systems have not been complete enough to achieve general use.

The initial hope that online interactive computers would have a major impact on medical education has not been realized. We doubt that this will change until specialty boards incorporate computers more completely into the examination process. Faculty believe that the curriculum is an important determinant of students' activities. The practical student focuses on passing examinations. The present examination system places a premium on memorized facts. A student receives no credit for knowing where information is stored or how to extract it from a computerized data bank. Given this somewhat discouraging picture, can we realistically predict a brighter future for information systems?

What Computers Can Do for Medical Practice in the Near Future

Inexpensive personal computers that can fit into any office put the practicing doctor in a position similar to that of the basic laboratory scientist who was given a LINC computer twenty years ago. Innovative uses of this new tool in medical practice, however, are developing at a slower pace than they did in the laboratory. The sources of support for basic scientists are more limited than those for the medical practice, and this makes the competition keener. The job of these scientists is creating, recording, analyzing, and publishing data leading to progress in the field of bioscience. They are involved personally in handling and manipulating data, and are willing to get involved with the computer.

Most doctors in practice do many things, and relegate office operation and data accumulation to the secretarial and technical staff. There is no need to analyze and change activities each day. These creatures of habit try to fit a computer into the practice in order to speed up or ease customary procedures. Other people put data into the computer and extract information from it. Such doctors miss the fact that material put in can be rearranged, and that the outputs can be of many kinds only loosely linked to inputs. The computer offers doctors a chance to develop new strategies and to change financial and medical records. When practicing physicians devote personal time and energy to using the computer in new ways, they can see real benefits.

This idea bears repeating: a computer can produce many different outputs if the data have been collected with more than one type of report in mind. If you are storing business-office procedure codes for established hypertension, a limited physical examination, and serum electrolytes, the computer can generate a bill for the visit and create utilization statistics for practice management, but the program can provide no medical data except that the patient has hypertension. If, on the other hand, the computer keeps a date of onset along with the diagnosis of hypertension, the actual results of the vital signs, funduscopic and cardiac examinations, and values for each electrolyte, an appropriate program can interpret the data to produce a variety of administrative or medical reports. After the initial entries are made, the computer can be updated rapidly by entering the values for items that change. Unchanged parameters can be carried forward automatically. The computer can summarize data or expand a report, depending on its purpose. Even if only abnormal physical findings have been recorded, the computer can generate a detailed executive physical examination, supplying pertinent negatives from a dictionary containing those parts of the examination the doctor always performs.

Doctors have routines they follow when a medical problem has been defined. In an encounter with acute illness, the computer can remind the doctor of the way in which he or she intends to handle the problem, and can note deviation from the routine. The computer can record the therapy and remind the doctor of a potential drug incompatibility. It can also remind the doctor of the date of the next visit, and generate instructions to prepare the patient for that visit.

A large part of any practice involves fairly standard prescriptions. These may be orders for single drugs on a short-term basis, or complex prescriptions for chemotherapy, dialysis, or nutrition schedules. The computer can decrease the time needed to initiate these schedules by physically printing the necessary documents, such as prescriptions, and by performing necessary mathematics such as adjusting an antibiotic dose for renal insufficiency.

In dealing with a chronic illness, the computer can create flow sheets to record needed information and to remind the doctor that it is time to collect new information. As data are recorded, the computer can tell whether there have been changes since the last entry, using the patient's own data as a control rather than using normal limits from a larger population.

Also, in a case of chronic illness, the computer can tell the doctor the findings at the first visit, the treatments undertaken, and the patient's current state. It allows the doctor to stratify patients with the same diagnosis into a set of subgroups. Outcome data can help determine the effectiveness of treatment. By gradually increasing the intervals between visits and tests in one portion of the practice, the doctor can determine optimal timing. The computer is like a time-lapse camera. It compresses time and allows the doctor to examine data from many patients over a period of years.

The computer can make life easier by managing appointments and scheduling. As diagnostic protocols are entered into the computer, scheduling algorithms optimize the use of all scarce resources, such as procedure rooms, and not just the doctor's time.

The computer can enhance business management in a practice. Charge capture and management of accounts receivable can be automated, reducing lost charges.

Computers are here. They are storing usable medical information, and the medical practice is slowly changing. As in most cases, the tortoise will out distance the hare. Those of us who are hares will have to develop patience.

IV

The Commumity and Doctors

We are a profession because we have adopted codes of ethics and have assumed service responsibilities not shared by the rest of society. Can these be maintained when the purpose of doctoring becomes the creating of profit for shareholders or the maintenance of expensive hospitals for the benefit of those who administer them but give no personal medical services?

Chapter 24

The Future Is Here

The future is here and we have done well by our patients. From the mid-1950s until 1968, age adjusted mortality remained constant and many critics of medicine believed that personal care given to patients by personal care doctors could relieve pain and suffering without affecting morbidity and mortality. Conventional wisdom stated that further decreases in age adjusted mortality would occur through changes in life style and not through application of biomedical knowledge developed by doctors, biomedical scientists and the pharmaceutical industry. Critics believe that the steadily rising cost of medical care given to individual patients could not be justified and should be scaled back.[1]

In 1972 a steady decline in age-adjusted death was noted which has continued year by year. We do know that conditions such as trauma, homicide, suicide, alcoholic cirrhosis—diseases most sensitive to social pathology—have not declined. Doctors have no leverage to cure poverty and illiteracy. They can only improve conditions when disease is the problem.

My own bias is that the steady decline in age-adjusted death rates that began in 1972 represents the cumulative effect of improvement in care of dozens of conditions that previously pro-

---

1. Stead EA, Jr. The Samuel L. Crow Lecture. Presented to the Area Health Education Center. Asheville, North Carolina, September 11, 1984.

duced dysfunction and incapacity to a degree that made financial independence and independent living difficult or impossible. Detailed study of these conditions would show improved function in individual patients but in no single study would the results be of a magnitude to change the age-adjusted death rate. My argument is strengthened by the fact that the downward slope of the curve of age-adjusted mortality that began in 1968 coincided with the implementation of Medicare and the Medicaid programs, which greatly increased the units of personal care given by doctors. What of the future? Our investment in bioscience of the last 35 years is just beginning to pay off. Golden years lie ahead. The doctors of tomorrow will have at their disposal an array of drugs, enzymes, hormones, synthetic materials, artificial systems and organs for transplantation that are unknown in my time. We are just unlocking the secrets of transforming agents that make somatic cells immortal. We will in time know the secret of ovum-sperm immortality. We will unlock the secret of aging before the year 2020. The mystery of memory and the ways to replenish the cells generating memory will be solved. Some new imaging techniques are here and many more are in the pipeline. We are learning the hard way the hazards of the workplace, but over the hill lie ways to make the body safer in hostile environments. I can think of no better time to be a bioscientist or a personal care doctor, using the output of science for the benefit of patients.

Without the statistical data to prove the point, practicing doctors have no doubt of the effectiveness of the personal health system in helping people survive more comfortably and live longer. They know that the use of available technology goes beyond that of any "Good Samaritan." They see a patient saved by a pacemaker or by control of ventricular tachycardia. They rejoice in the graduation from the Harvard Medical School of a person with childhood leukemia, a fatal disease in the not-too-distant past. They play golf with a previously crippled friend freed from inactivity by bilateral hip replacement. They have a leading basketball player who performs because of the effectiveness of bronchodilator drugs. Their bridge-playing patient is back in tournament competition because of a drug that blocks the secretion of hydrochloric acid by the stomach. Their patients with angina have increased their exercise tolerance by the use of a series of drugs introduced in the last 15 years. They rarely see malignant hypertension and when they do it is no longer the killer of old. Steroid therapy makes living tolerable for many persons. Acute lupus erythematosus is now controllable; there are many non-steroidal anti-inflammatory drugs that increase the. range of activities of patients with arthritis. The notion of statistical measurements to justify the technology seems absurd to personal care doctors. They see the before and the after very clearly. They have not cured disease but they have postponed illness, and his patients are no longer incapacitated.

The cumulative effects of medical care, each increasing life expectancy and reduced morbidity in some areas, eventually reached a magnitude to bring the curve of age-adjusted mortality in line with the perception of the doctor. From 1970 to 1975 death rates dropped 14%—from 747 to 642 persons a year in a population of 100,000. This rate of decline is equal to any seen in this century and has continued to the present. Mortality has decreased in ten of the fifteen major causes of death.

To make this scenario come true we need doctors. Many things can be said about personal health services but the most important single fact is that they cannot be given without doctors. We can control our fate if we make correct choices.

Before 1937 the practice of medicine was carried on mostly in doctors' offices. The era of modern technology was just evolving. X-ray units were housed in basements and there were no skilled chemists in the clinical laboratories. Doctors were kindly and considerate but rarely life-saving. It took many years to establish the economic base for a successful practice. With the advent of sulfanilimide doctors became much more useful. A multitude of technical advances allowed each doctor to care for many more patients. The economic base of medicine grew rapidly and doctors began to develop habits of practice that allowed them to be more efficient. They gave up house calls and concentrated their work in hospitals and offices. Group practice and specialization grew apace. Doctors entering practice were assured an excellent income from Day 1. Doctors worked long hours for their economic rewards. Under pressure they increasingly structured their working environment to meet their own needs. Insurance paid for by government or by industry poured money into the system. The doctors being well paid did not oppose the growth of the hospital. They became more and more dependent on the help supplied by the hospital. The patients followed the lead of the doctors. Insurance companies and industry were there for the convenience of the doctor.

By the 1980s troubles began to brew. In the 1960s and 1970s third-party payers were protected by the number of hospital beds. Because most covered services were given in hospitals, maximum costs could be calculated and the premium adjusted accordingly. Third party payers wanted to lower cost. The public was not willing to decrease the amount of care.

We all know that the hospitals and nursing homes get most of the health care dollars. Experiences of prepaid medical groups have uniformly shown that medical expenses are lowered when the doctor is rewarded financially for a reduction in cost. To date the decrease in cost has been produced by hospitalizing fewer patients and by reducing the length of stay. It is hoped that the share of health dollars going to nursing homes will be reduced in a variety of ways by keeping patients out of nursing homes and making medical technology mobile enough to be used in the home. For-profit and not-for-profit organizations, governmental agencies, and community agencies are entering the home health care arena with mobile technologies that can be used in homes caring for one to four patients. On August 20, 1984, Duke announced home health care services for the following procedures: total parenteral nutrition, intravenous antibiotic services, internal feeding service, chemotherapy service. In this same month Durham County Hospital Corporation was licensed to give home health care. It is too early to determine to what extent nursing home costs will be reduced. In areas where these programs are very active, there is to date a noticeable decrease in pressure on nursing home beds.

There is plenty of money at the level of 10% of Gross National Product to support the doctors who are going into practice. Remember that between 1980 and 1983 the work force increased by five million. The Gross National Product increased by 99 billion dollars over the same period. Ten percent of this figure is 9.9 billion, or a 3.3 billion dollar increase for medical services each year. No one expects the total medical bills to decline. It is predicted that medical expenses will retain their current relationship to the Gross National Product and that inflation will be reduced to the level present in the rest of the economy. That means there are lots of dollars to be played with. The name of the game will be who gets the dollars.

Doctors have to decide to what degree they wish the health care dollar to be spent by large corporations that control for-profit hospitals and nursing homes and by hospitals with large debts to bondholders. It is clear that the more dollars that go into these units the less dollars to the doctors and the more impersonal the services to the patient. We are at the crossroads. We are a profession because we have adopted codes of ethics and have assumed service responsibilities not shared by the rest of society. Can these be maintained when the purpose of doctoring becomes the creating of profit for shareholders or the maintenance of expensive hospitals for the benefit of those who administer them but give no personal medical services?

The movement of women into the work force, the disappearance of domestic help, and the aging of our population have created situations where organizations of some sort have to supply and coordinate services to allow wage earners to continue to work. These services have to be supplied by hospitalization, by admission to nursing homes, or by organizations capable of supplying services on an ambulatory basis in holding areas related to the doctor's office, in small rest homes, in day care centers and homes.

For-profit organizations supplying home health care services and temporary nursing services are a rapidly growing industry. Hospitals are applying for licenses to operate these services. Ambulatory surgicenters and free-standing emergency centers are being franchised on a national basis or operated by hospitals or groups of doctors. In the Minneapolis-St. Paul area there are health maintenance organizations and seven ambulatory surgical centers. Hospital occupancy had decreased to 60%. A 39-day nurses' strike had further accelerated the decline in occupancy and increased the amount of care given in surgicenters and by home care agencies. Hospital patients were discharged earlier and seen by visiting nurses at home. The hospitals and ambulatory surgery centers increased the number of operations done on an outpatient basis. Sicker patients were sent home to be cared for by organizations selling temporary nursing services. Coronary angiograms were performed on an outpatient basis. An investigation by the Minnesota Department of Health and Human Services found that patients' health was not jeopardized by the strike. Once the doctors discovered that the hospital could not serve their patients in the traditional way, they devised satisfactory and cheaper substitutes for the hotel services the hospital had traditionally supplied. Most observers of the Minneapolis - St. Paul scene believe that these changes initiated by the nurses strike will not be reversed. There will be a permanent redistribution of the health care dollar with the hospital share decreasing.

What will be the role of doctors as the bed component of hospitals decreases and more work is done in ambulatory settings? Will there be a shift of the hospital's share of the money to agencies operated by hospitals and by franchised health services or will the doctors band together to supply the manpower to care for their patients in non-hospital and non-nursing-home settings? Will we use a part of the output of our medical schools to produce doctors who can manage these decentralized units?

In 1971 I discussed the advantages of diversifying the education of a portion of our medical students to provide a steady stream of physician managers.

Medical schools are just now facing up to the fact that they need physicians trained in both management and medicine. When we say that premedical education should include more of the information sciences, business administration, economics, sociology and systems engineering we are not thinking of the traditional physician, but we are expressing our conviction that we need managing physicians.

My prediction is that doctors will organize groups that are capable of providing a wide range of professional services to their patients with minimal use of the hospital. I see group practices with 10 holding beds for short-term stays in their clinics and an arrangement with a nearby motel for minimal care to cover patient stays for up to three weeks. Most of the care will be in the patient's home or in small or convalescent homes where one to five patients may be housed, the personnel to service these units — clinic beds, motel coverage, homes, and convalescent homes — will be supplied by the group practice. Money traditionally going to the hospital with its high capital costs and high overhead will flow into new channels.

Major changes are coming in the organization of x-ray and laboratory services. Traditionally, practicing radiologists have been essential because they had to spend years learning to read the gray scales of conventional radiography. Digital subtraction techniques will give black and white images that are simple to interpret. The images will have the black and white aspects that we now find in a good clean broken bone. Anyone can read that x-ray and it does not require the training and years of experience to read the image. X-ray will move out of the hospital and back into the doctor's office. The new equipment will be more complicated to maintain and the persons maintaining the equipment will become more important than the person interpreting the images.

The clinical laboratory will came closer to the patient. Small, portable units with computerized output will supply the doctor with on-line data and the need for follow-up visits to review the data from the laboratory will be greatly decreased. Home kits for diagnosis and portable treatments will proliferate. Home kits to test for pregnancy are already in common use.

Medical equipment businesses are providing the equipment for office and home use. Diagnostic equipment designed for use outside hospitals will have sales of 350 million dollars by 1985 and could pass one billion dollars by 1990. Five percent of all blood analysis is done in the offices of doctors. In-office testing will be a common way to generate income. It is predicted that new, smaller and cheaper diagnostic units, having fewer moving parts, lower maintenance costs and operated by less skilled personnel will capture 25% of the testing market. The time between testing and delivery of the results will be reduced to minutes. There will be no need for a follow-up visit to review the laboratory data.

Home dialysis for kidney patients has taught us a lot. It is now clear that an uncomplicated patient with bacterial endocarditis does not need to be treated in a hospital. A newly discovered diabetic does not require hospitalization for education and regulation. Most cancer chemotherapy can be given without hospitalization. The hospital will be used for sophisticated surgery: neurosurgery, transplants, implantation of artificial organs, reconstructive creation and modification of life, high-risk deliveries and trauma. Most postoperative care will be given outside the hospital.

The shift of care away from the hospital requires that patients be taught how to assume more responsibility for their care. Home dialysis has taught us that home care is practical if the patient becomes less mystified by procedures and more willing to take responsibility. Home monitoring of blood sugar levels has emphasized the same thing. Doctors will give episodic care to patients without engaging in patient education. They will include patient education as a part of the clinic's program when caring for patients with chronic illness.

My forecast for the future is a pluralistic system in which medical care will be given by doctors working for hospitals and for-profit organizations and by doctors running more complex group practices structured towards ambulatory care with minimal use of the hospital. Group practices will be interrelated for the purposes of training personnel at all levels to supply a full range of ambulatory services and to purchase capital intensive equipment requiring skilled personnel for maintenance.

Any unit with an investment in expensive technology will operate at night and on weekends. The transfer of basic science knowledge to new areas of practices, more woman doctors with a shorter work week, and more doctors to do functions previously carried out in the hospital, will keep all of us busy. I'm not one who believes that there will be an oversupply of doctors once we change our ways.

Most of our prophets predict that we will have too many doctors. There will be a significant increase in the number of doctors per 1,000 persons. Because of the movement of women into the labor forces the ratio of number of doctors to the number of workers will rise more slowly. With money to pay them obtained by regaining a portion of dollars presently spent by hospital and nursing homes, the doctors will remain busy. Specialization has always been the cutting edge of medicine and it will continue to be in the future. Doctors are going to have to demonstrate that what they do makes a difference and this something must be something one cannot do without the education and skill of the doctor. I believe that we will have too many generalists. Their field is going to be continually narrowed by the specialists who will contend that all poor outcomes would have been avoided if the patients had had specialist skills at their disposal. In this era of easy travel and free communications the courts are going to require that each doctor perform at the best national level and not at the level present in his community. There will be too much overlap between the activities of the generalist and those of allied health professionals and nurses. My advice to young doctors is to enjoy their years of preparation for practice and to specialize to a degree where only doctors can compete. Doctors and hospital administrators need to alert each other about their plans for the future. Hospitals need to know that plans are afoot to use them less. They will need time for necessary adjustments.

In my day, medicine has been a profession. A profession is characterized by a code of ethics enforced by its members. The code of ethics for a profession must require of its members behavior of benefit to society of a nature not expected from non-professionals. Medicine is a service profession and traditionally requires of its members 24-hour service to people who are ill and frequently distraught, irrational, and hostile. It is this requirement of service given willingly and skillfully at all times and to all people that separates our profession from occupations that require an investment in education and apprenticeship equal to that of the doctor. The heads of our large corporations, ship captains, makers of steel, computer experts are very skilled operators but we do not say that they belong to a profession. They are intelligent persons responding in our society primarily to the profit motive.

Today I see many non-professional doctors in practice. A few weeks ago on a Sunday, one of my neighbors, 55 miles away from his home, had a small stroke. He asked me to talk to his wife and call his doctor. He had a history of hypertension and atrial fibrillation. I did call his doctor because of the possibility of an embolus from his left atrium. The doctor, who was the only one of his group of four who knew the patient, declined to talk on the telephone with my neighbor and referred him to his colleague. The colleague arranged for him to telephone on Monday morning and make an appointment with the doctor who had refused to talk with him on Sunday. The appointment wars for the following Friday at which time coumadin was started. I believe that doctors who practice this way are not members of a profession. Either coumadin was not indicated or it should have been started immediately with coverage by heparin for the first three days. This doctor was certainly not a member of the medical profession. I doubt that you could even call him a skilled craftsman.

I believe it is easier to preserve the professional ethic if doctors can run their own affairs. My illustration shows that it does not always work that way. The prospect of doctors running large ambulatory and clinic services reminds us of the old days when one or two doctors ran for-profit, proprietary hospitals. Our hope is that better educated doctors and better educated patients will avoid the conflict of interest very clearly seen in doctor-operated proprietary hospitals of the past. Only time will tell.

Regardless of who runs the show there will be major changes in the small Hill-Burton hospitals in North Carolina. They have too many acute care beds and too little nursing and home care facilities. They do need to have their accommodations updated to at least compete with a good motel. They need fewer beds, a wider range of specialists, less investment in any expensive equipment not fully used, and a working relationship with a tertiary hospital.[2]

---

2. Two papers from which Dr. Stead drew information in this essay are: Paul Starr, *The Social Transformation of American Medicine*. New York: Basic Books, Inc./Rarper Colophon Books, 1982, pp. 409-10, and Douglas Henderson-James, *Technological Change and Rural Hospital Survival*. Delivered to the Rowland Health Planning Seminar, Duke Endowment, Charlotte, North Carolina, July 8-10, 1984.

Chapter 25

On Community Hospitals

M any questions are being raised in medical circles about the development of the educational programs in community hospitals.[1] I would like you to know my thoughts.

Educational programs in community hospitals are rarely successful. They are commonly modeled after university medical centers. Because the functions and financing of the university medical center and the community hospital are widely different, it is not surprising that the transplanted program does not flourish in the new environment.

The medical center receives funds to support the time that the faculty spends in teaching and training. It also supports the time the faculty spends in the laboratory and library preparing for its teaching duties. The university medical center can, therefore, make the expensive investment in time required for converting untrained personnel into a highly skilled product.

The community hospital is a user of the skilled personnel produced by the university medical center. The professional staff of the community hospital gives service to the community. The demands for service are so great that the physician has little time for contemplation and postgraduate education. Any program of training or teaching put into the community hospital which requires an investment of professional time makes matters worse.

1. Stead EA, Jr. A letter to Dr. Barnes Woodhall, Dean of Duke University School of Medicine, June 18, 1965.

The last bits of thinking time disappear with the assumption of additional teaching. A teaching service is added to an already heavy patient-service load.

It is not surprising that community hospital educational programs falter when they attempt to teach new classes of interns and residents each year. With a great effort, the staff spends time with the residents only to discover that they do this at the expense of their last leisure moments. They do not have the time both to prepare for their teaching activities and then to perform them.

The key problem is how to return some free time for thinking to the professional staff of the community hospital. The traditional program of adding interns and residents will fail, in general, for the reasons outlined above. There is a second reason why such programs modeled on the medical center will not be widely successful. There are not enough interns and residents produced to staff the majority of community hospitals. One can set up a program which robs Peter to pay Paul, but it is not possible to pay both Peter and Paul. Doctors have added a new profession--one selected by doctors, educated by doctors and employed by doctors. These persons are called physician-assistants or associates and will replace interns and residents in most community hospitals.

Accepting the premises that (1) continuing postgraduate education is an advantage to the physician, the hospital and community, (2) transplantation of the educational and training functions of the university medical center based on a large faculty with the time for teaching green personnel will not work in the community hospital, and (3) the key problem is to free up time for the professional staff so that they can read, arrange conferences, and think—what can be done?

1.   The hospital can be planned with a view to conserv-

ing the time of the physician and allowing him to continue his education. Good community hospital planning should include:

a. conference and assembly rooms
b. a clinic building to house the offices of its staff
c. central chemistry laboratory under a chemist's direction to do all clinic and hospital work
d. adequate general laboratory under the direction of a pathologist
e. a place for teaching in the x-ray department
f. a library with current journals and a good tie-in with a regional library connected with the National Library of Medicine. This library would have taped material as well as books; it would have a recording of the major conferences of at least one medical center.

2. A geographical full-time professional staff to advise the hospital administrator on ways to save staff time. This staff should be supported in part by the hospital and in part by money contributed by the professional staff for the educational program. There should be, at a minimum, a representative from each of the major clinical departments. Only a portion of each doctor's time would be supported by the budget. The remainder would be created by practice. This group would be the catalyst to stimulate the professional staff to use for educational purposes the leisure time created. The entire staff would participate in the reading, the thinking, and the preparation of the conferences. The professional staff would participate in the educational program in the role of teacher and student.

3. The professional staff would include specialists in all

the major areas of clinical specialization. Consultation fees would be held at a low level so that every difficult problem would present an opportunity for real graduate education.

4. The heads of the clinical departments would be responsible for devising ways to use the doctor's time more effectively. They would identify personnel capable of organizing the health services given under the direction of the doctors. These personnel would perform many of the duties in the community hospital that, in the university medical center, are done by interns and residents. They would form a cadre of top assistants who could direct, under the doctor's direction, health care in the clinic, in the hospital, and in the home. In my opinion, no satisfactory postgraduate programs applicable on a state-wide basis will be successful until these new physician-assistants are trained and actively at work. They can create for the physician the needed ingredient: time.

In summary, I have a great interest in developing new programs and patterns in community hospitals. I have no interest at all in attempting to shore up existing programs that I believe are certain to fail. Current programs based on employing an educational director, with the anticipation that he can create time for the staff by an influx of interns and residents, are not based on sound thinking. They do not identify the essential missing ingredient: thinking time for the staff.[2]

---

2. In 1965 Gene Stead began the Physician Assistants Program. This memo was an early communication about the program to the Dean of Duke Medical School. See Chapters 28-32 on the role of physician extenders in health care.

Chapter 26

The Assets of a Community Hospital

A university medical center is a place where raw manpower is converted into trained manpower. It uses the familiar areas of teaching, research, and service to produce this trained manpower.[1]

A community hospital is one where trained manpower gives health services to members of the community. The community hospital has many advantages in providing health services if it clearly defines its role and does not attempt to become a primary manpower converting system.

A community hospital staffed with the output of the university residency programs has a tremendous teaching potential. The residents have devoted many years to the interrelated processes of learning and teaching. Every chief resident that I trained has had much more formal teaching experience than the majority of the instructors that teach my children in college. Every doctor trained in depth in any subspecialty has had an equally long background in the educational system.

We have always emphasized the need for the resident-in-training to be active in the learning processes of others because information transfer and the stimulation of the patient to learn are the bread and butter of most medical practice. This potential

---

1. Stead EA, Jr. The assets of a community hospital. *Medical Times*, 97:225-226, 1969.

educational wealth within its staff has not been tapped to the fullest by community hospitals. It is a resource that must be used if we are going to allow workers in the health field to develop their own full potential.

The physician in a community hospital will find that the retraining of raw manpower each year is expensive in time and money. The effort will remove the last vestiges of time from his already busy day. If, on the other hand, he begins to devote his energies to training a stable group of people who will remain active for many years in the care of his patients in the home, the office and the hospital, he will have a different experience. This approach will return time to the hard-pressed doctor.

I know of no instance in which the expense of an intern and residency program in a community hospital has been accurately cost-accounted. The current rise in pay to interns and residents will cause some hospitals to collect these data. Attention must be given to the cost of the inefficiencies inherent in the manpower converting system and the high cost of retraining. My own bias is obvious. I'd run my community hospital on trained manpower rather than on raw manpower. I'd use the teaching potential of my staff to develop a permanent, competent, supporting staff. I'd put more time—not less—in my own day.

Chapter 27

Picking Other People's Brains

P lanning becomes essential to a venture when the venture requires the expenditure of a large amount of capital; when there is a long lag time between the commitment of the capital and the first sale or use of the product; when the products to be produced are so specialized that they can be used effectively for only one purpose; and when the capital available is insufficient to produce all possible products and, therefore, the course of action selected prevents other courses of action from being pursued with great intensity.[1]

I grew up in the era when the capital available to the educational and health ventures was small; when the time devoted to education was short; when the educational and health fields were directed by and in turn produced generalists. Then educational and health organizations grew by simple additions to existing systems. The definition of goals, the analysis of the alternate paths that might be trod to reach the goals, the cost effectiveness of a series of possible programs, the annual production of a five-year projection of our program, the advantages to be gained by a continuous synthesis of highly individualistic programs, were foreign to our thinking. Universities, the health professions and medical centers did not have the staff to collect the information necessary to make crucial decisions involving alternate methods

1. Stead EA, Jr. Picking other people's brains. *Medical Times*, 97:264–266, 1969.

of operation. Indeed, the need for such staff was rarely recognized.

I have never ceased to be astonished at how easy it is to be wise about other people's affairs and how difficult it is to be wise about one's own. We were all critical of the old procedure of fixing an arbitrary national budget for national defense and then apportioning this budget among the various services in the absence of a single, approved plan for the defense department, projected far enough into the future to insure that all programs were both possible and desirable. With the shoe on the other foot, however, we became immediately defensive if the development of a long-range plan in our medical center did not begin with the statement that any new plan would not reduce existing budgets or limit the existing prerogatives of any chairman.

Anyone interested in planning will profit by reading Mr. McNamara's account[2] of his approach to planning and budgeting for the defense establishment. He notes that the authority for management of the Department of Defense was present when he became Secretary, but that efficient machinery to allow the Secretary of Defense to exercise this authority was lacking. Robert McNamara said: "The problem may be considered this way: in order to make crucial decisions on force levels and weapons, the President, the Secretary of Defense and Congress must have complete information focused on those questions and their place in the over-all military system. They need to know, for example, the military effectiveness and the cost of a B-52 squadron as it relates to a Minuteman missile squadron and a Polaris submarine. The data must include not only the cost of equipping these units but also the cost of manning and operating them for various periods. Only under these circumstances can the alternatives be

---

2. McNamara RS. *The Essence of Being a Secretary, Reflections in Office.* New York: Harper and Row, Publishers Inc., 1968.

made fully clear."

"One of the first things we did in 1961 was to design a new mechanism which would provide this information and integrate it into a single, coherent management system. The product of this effort was the Planning-Programming-Budgeting System, which is now being widely applied throughout the U.S. Government and which is being introduced in foreign governments as well.

"For the Defense Department, this system serves several very important purposes:

1. It provides the mechanism through which financial budgets, weapons programs, force requirements, military strategy and foreign policy objectives are all brought into balance with one another.
2. It produces the annual Five-Year Defense Program, which is perhaps the most important single management tool for the Secretary of Defense and the basis for the annual proposal to Congress.
3. It permits the top management of the Defense Department, the President and the Congress to focus their attention on the tasks and missions related to our national objectives rather than on the tasks and missions of a particular service.
4. It provides for the entire Defense Establishment a single approved plan, projected far enough into the future to ensure that all the programs are both physically and financially feasible."

The same problems outlined by Mr. McNamara are present in every university and medical center. As the health field develops new mixes of manpower and machines, our capital costs will rise, the time between initiation of programs and their pay-off in

better health will increase, our manpower will be more specialized and among the many possible in lines of development a few
will have to be selected. Clearly, we cannot afford to disregard
the lessons to be learned from ventures in planning which have
been carried out in other segments of our society.

V

The Medical Workforce: Some New Ideas

T he question of what physician's assistants should do is one we have not tried to determine. It is perfectly clear that the economics of the situation require that they must do some of the things a doctor has done traditionally. They cannot be used for convenience, just to make life a little easier for the doctor. They have to do things the doctor did and to be paid for them; the doctor must then do other things, or there is no worth in this system.

Chapter 28

Educational Programs and Manpower

I live in a medical school, and therefore my points of reference are the educational programs that supply manpower for the health field.[1] There is a difference between the university whose function is to take green manpower and turn out trained manpower and the health service unit whose function is to give health services with the use of trained manpower. A manpower-converting unit is not the most efficient research unit or the most efficient service unit. A university does research and takes care of sick people in order to develop manpower. We do not do research as a primary interest. Our output is man. We do not give medical services as a primary interest. Our output again is man. For the production of the manpower we do use both the tools of research and the tools of medical care and its implementation.

May I point out that the educational field is of necessity inefficient? One can never educate anyone to think if at the same time one is requiring him to have maximal efficiency in the use of those things that he has already learned. Education is essentially putting bits of information into pupils' heads and then giving them the opportunity and the chance to build new structures, to make new things and, above all, to make mistakes. So, an educational institution by its very nature is an inefficient insti-

---

1. Stead EA, Jr. Educational programs and manpower. *Bull. N.Y. Acad. Med.*, 44:204-213, 1968.

tution. In the clinical training of manpower, it must remain in part inefficient in regard even to use of technical, secretarial, and other kinds of help—for the very real reason that it is not desirable to raise the basic cost of the unit in which the physician is getting his education to the point where it must produce the maximal amount of services. If this happens, it is not possible to carry out the education. It is unfortunate that most of our physicians and nurses go into areas set up primarily for service, where their only experience has been a rather long one in manpower-converting units. When they start to function in what are primarily service roles, they begin, of course, to attempt to create in their service functions exactly what they had in the manpower-converting units. And many of the problems that relate to the organization of health care, particularly in community hospitals, relate to this frame of reference, which is really, I think, no longer a very good frame of reference when the giving of services is the primary goal.

I believe the time has come for the university system to begin to set up opportunities for an individual who has completed his training to work in an area that is concerned primarily with the effective use of trained manpower to give health care. This unit will be a user of trained manpower, not a producer of trained manpower. The university will need to agree to produce any type of manpower needed by the service area.

In order to do this, of course, one must have money, personnel, and ability. Duke University has given some consideration to this matter. I shall describe these things because I do not know any other way to be useful to you except to tell you what we are doing. We decided that we cannot produce manpower and illustrate the proper use of manpower for health services within the existing university unit. We simply cannot make the service unit a primary goal and function in the middle of a manpower-converting unit and have it make sense.

So we are going a distance away from the hospital and, under the direction of Dr. Harvey Estes, chairman of our Department of Community Health Services, we are setting up a new building complex. We are going to set up a new faculty and a new fiscal organization, with monies-whatever is accumulated for this venture-to feed back into the business. Except for raising the money, I think that the planning has gone pretty well. And it will be a few years before we know whether there is any wisdom in this approach to the matter. I should like to say a word about the names in the health profession which do get us into trouble. People look on a physician with an M.D. as a sort of uniform product, when actually M.D.'s are no longer interchangeable. Physicians have a very wide spectrum of activities, and therefore the determination of how many doctors there are in relation to population gives you no information about the number of persons available for any particular kind of work that physicians do.

We are in even worse trouble in regard to nurses. If one uses the word "nurse" the term gives a fairly uniform picture to the physician and to many of the consumers of health care. But, interestingly enough, this picture is quite different from the picture the word "nurse" conveys to the nursing educator. We should have to say, at least in our part of the world, that nursing education is becoming a general form of education. Students are fun to talk to and to work with; they generally marry well and they live well. But they are no longer a very active force in the field of health. And, because of the amount of time that is devoted to general education in the course of the relatively short half-life of active work in the field, we no longer look upon a nurse primarily as a person allied with the physician who is going to give care in the field of health. We must begin to bring into the field of health persons more closely allied with it who will, on a career basis, stay with it longer. So, as the whole world changes around us, we are even tripped up by the use of names.

It is interesting, as a problem in communication and learning, to see nurse educators talk to a group of doctors and explain to them that their goal is a general education not closely related to activities in the hospital. Two or three weeks later, ask a group of doctors to give you the gist of what was said. The doctors never remember being told that the hospital is no longer the central point in nurses training. But I think the educator of the nurse has a point, and I think we had better pay attention to it. We are living in a time when new professionals are going to have to be brought into the health field if the physician is to find it possible to discharge his duties. Let me draw a parallel again with the nursing field. About 20 years ago it became obvious that there were not going to be enough nurses to fill the requirements of the field of health. But it was difficult to establish general appreciation of this eventuality and it was difficult to initiate programs that would eventually take up the slack in the nursing field.

The problem seems highlighted to me by the fact that the nurse in our hospital is the only person who cannot learn. Anyone else in the hospital can be upgraded in their work because they have time to learn something new every year. But our nurses have reached the point where they are in such short supply and are so overcome by their responsibilities that they have no time for learning.

This is the same point that is beginning to confront the physician. If you watch the average physician in practice, you discover that they now have little time for learning. As we attempt to give medical care to the entire population, our current supply of physicians is not going to suffice. Unless we begin to add more workers to the health field, physicians will find themselves within the next 10 to 15 years in exactly the situation in which nurses are now. And for all I know, they may use the same solution—namely, withdraw as a major factor in the health field.

We do have a difference in point of view between those people who believe the past can be recreated and shored up by tinkering with it here or there, and those individuals who believe that a new era is beginning, that an old era is ended, and that not too much time should be spent in tinkering with or shoring up the past. It seems clear to me that one era is ended and that another has begun.

I should like to say a few words about the problem of putting doctors in relation to persons who in the past have not received medical care. I was certainly a slow learner in this area. It is easy for one to learn something in one field and find it difficult to relate it to other fields in which one is less active.

For years we have been concerned with the problem of what to do with persons who have come from countries that have a much less well-developed society than we have and a much less developed educational system than we have. Frequently they come to this country for college, where they spend four years. They go through four years of medical school. Then they go through four or five years of professional training in this country. When they return home they find a society into which they cannot fit and find no niche in which they can be useful. Having made a large emotional commitment to one way of life, with 1-2 years of fairly hard work, they tend either to be unhappy where they are or to return here.

We now wish to give modern medical care to a large section of our population who have received limited care in the past. We have the question of how do we get doctors to them. And it is becoming obvious to us that those bright African American students who compete well in colleges, who get into Harvard Medical School, and who come to Duke University for four years of postgraduate training are not of any help to us in this problem. And we are dealing with exactly the same kind of situation that confronted us when we took other persons out of their culture or changed their culture for 12 years and then wished them to return to it. So we have begun the slow process of identifying persons who have never lost their contact with the culture we need to help. Under the leadership of Dr. Charles D. Watts,[2] a program has been established at Lincoln Hospital, Durham, N.C., to train graduates of Meharry Medical College and also of Howard University. These students use the facilities of Duke Medical Center to receive training at Lincoln. Part of the time is spent at Duke Medical Center. On graduation from the training program, the doctors join the medical clinic of Lincoln Hospital and take care of both public and private patients. This has converted a totally charitable and somewhat dilapidated operation into one that is creating money and new jobs in Durham.

Such developments take time. They also take willingness on our part to arrange instructions somewhat differently than we do for our usual graduates, but we have been pleased with our results. We are not training second-class physicians. We are training physicians in a different way, in a different pattern of time, and we are allowing them to begin to create income from practice at a much earlier date than their counterparts do in a different social setting, and we are taking somewhat longer in certain phases of that training.

We are not training scientists, but we are attempting to train doctors who will relate to a community that never before has had medical services. We are beginning to get physicians to

---

2. Charles D. Watts is a pioneer of medicine in Durham, NC. He has been a key leader in Durham for many years advocating for access to health care for all members of the Durham community and for creating and sustaining Durham's reputation as the "City of Medicine." Dr. Watts helped integrate Lincoln and Watts Hospitals into Durham Regional Hospital in Durham, and established the Lincoln Community Health Center to serve Durham residents without medical insurance.

cover an area of our population with good medical care, which they have never received before.

In attempting to improve the ability of a doctor to give more services, we have begun to look at the question of how he should be supplied with assistants. We have attempted to separate the things the physician does that require judgment from those that require some intelligence and some skill and that are recycled every day. And, as you analyze the activities of the physician in this way, it becomes obvious that many things that have been done traditionally by doctors can be done by non-doctors. We are also confronted with the fact that, at this time in history, specialization is with us, and that it is now very difficult for the hospital to produce personnel trained to fit the many needs of the various kinds and aspects of medical practice. It seemed to us that the physician had to define what his needs were, had to find the population that could serve those needs, and had to train persons selected from it to act as helpers.

So, beginning on an informal basis four years ago,[3] and on a rather formal basis two years ago, we have begun to train a group of persons whom we have elected to call physician's assistants and that is exactly what they are. These are persons recruited by the doctors; they are trained by the doctor; and in the end we intend them to be paid by the doctor.

Of course, we have had the problems that one would expect to find in any new field. We have had the question from nurses as to whether we were stealing things that belonged to them. We have had questions from our own interns, from our resident staff, and from our senior professional staff. Were we going to get in trouble by having people do things done traditionally by physicians? Would the assistants eventually set up as doctors? We have had trouble from hospital administrators who would like to

---

3. "Four years ago" refers to 1964.

remain in complete command from the nursing service up to the hospital superintendent. Administrators have wanted the duties and the financial rewards of this particular group of persons to be determined by hospital management rather than by doctors. We have had trouble with government officials in looking for support because they have said that, in order to work in the field of health at any advanced level, a college degree is necessary. Having been to college myself, I have always been a little skeptical about this requirement. More than a college education, one needs dedication to the field of health and a willingness to give service, some understanding of why sick persons are irrational, and why patients make demands that well people do not make.

Each year the physician's assistant can learn things he did not know the year before. The assistant must feel that he has made a lifetime commitment. He does not work a few years and stop, then another few years and stop; he says, "This is my business," and he works at it year in and year out. In the students we have selected for training, the turn of the social wheel has been such that they have gone only through high school and are not financially in a position to go to college. I do not think anything would be gained by sending these students to college for four years when they have shown that they want to be in the health field and are ready to go to work. So we have been in the awkward position of being willing to take high school graduates. The supporting agencies would not object to this if we were to give them a very short course. But we are giving them a two-year course that does have in it considerable individualization and is relatively expensive per student. There is plenty of money available to give short courses to high school graduates and long courses to college graduates, but we have had trouble in obtaining funds for a two-year course for high school graduates.

This is an extraordinarily complex nation. North Carolina is very unlike New York City. It is very unlike Montana. I do not think for a minute that the pattern we are setting up of turning high school graduates into physician's assistants is a pattern recommended for the entire country. I should like to see someone start this program at the college level in order to find out what characteristics persons would have who remained longer in the field of health and what various capabilities they would develop. Since an old system is ending, we all ought to be testing new programs that are feasible in our own respective areas.

The question of what a physician's assistant should do is one we have not tried to determine. It is perfectly clear that the economics of the situation require that he must do some of the things a doctor has done traditionally. He cannot be used for convenience, just to make life a little easier for the doctor. He has to do things the doctor did and to be paid for them; the doctor must then do other things, or there is no worth in this system.

The point we come to immediately is that physicians must be trained along with physician's assistants; otherwise they really do not know how to use them and what to do with them. Our general plan was for physician's assitant students to have a year of didactic work supervised by the persons with whom they will work. We did not want to farm out biochemistry to the biochemist. We wanted the physician to teach that part of biochemistry that is relevant to current medical practice. Physician's assistants have no trouble in determining pH and, statistically, they can move hydrogen ions about the body as well as a doctor three years out of medical school can. We have wished assistants to have some general knowledge of pharmacology but we have not wanted them taught by the pharmacologist. They are taught by physicians who are interested in therapy and the use of drugs, who determine the content of pharmacology. All our doctors have not liked this because they must take the time to do the teaching. It is always easier if somebody else will do the teaching, but this training would have a different quality. The subjects covered in the first year are the same as those covered in medical school. They are given from a different viewpoint. The second year, we put the assistant in those areas of the hospital that have a high doctor-patient ratio. These include the emergency clinic, the admission room at the Veterans Administration Hospital, the recovery room, the respiratory care unit, the endocrine clinic, the cardiac care unit, and group and individual practices in the state prison hospitals of North Carolina.

Medical care is a continuum. What one does depends on how much effort one wants to spend in learning. A nurse does nothing different from a doctor; a professional nurse does everything a nonprofessional does but has additional duties. A student who devotes four years to training will do somewhat less than a student who devotes six years to training. But there is no magic in the system. It depends on the time commitment one wants to make, the time one wants to put in before one actually is administering health care on a service basis.

So, all these things can be taught. One progressively can be responsible for a larger area. We don't have a good system of vertical movement in the health field. I am certainly not in a position to throw stones at anybody. The medical profession is as rigid as any other part of this system. A physician's assistant should be able to do anything that continuously recycles.

Chapter 29

Training and Use of Paramedical Personnel

T he doctor is the person licensed by the state to diagnose and treat disease. He has always had helpers: nurses, administrators, technicians, physiotherapists, dietitians and social workers.[1] These persons have been responsible for facilitating the arrangements for the flow of patients, for meeting the physical needs of sick people and for carrying out, under his direction, a variety of examinations and treatments. In most states, the doctors, registered nurses and practical nurses are the only licensed members of the health team.

The healthcare team has not been structured to allow free movement among the various classes of workers. Qualifying as a practical nurse does not make it much easier to become a registered nurse. Registered nurses from a diploma school do not receive much credit if they wish to graduate from a nursing school that awards a college degree. Excellent nurses with a large amount of experience with patients receive little credit if they wish to enroll in medical school. The non-physician complement of the health areas has been related to institutions or to administration, and often has not shared in the real excitement of the venture. Most of the satisfactions of the health field come from working with the patients and sharing in the emotional

---

1. Stead EA, Jr. Medical intelligence: Current concepts. Training and use of paramedical personnel. *N. Eng. J. Med.*, 277:800-801, 1967.

rewards that come from service effectively rendered to the individual person. Doctors are in a position to share these rewards with the rest of the health team. If they do, they are very effective recruiters and trainers. If they do not, they will have few capable helpers.

Health services to the individual patient extend from the person who first receives the telephone call about the patient, or who first registers him, up through the more esoteric specialist. There is no sharp break in the services rendered by the receptionist, the orderly, the nurse's aide, the practical nurse, the registered nurse, the professional nurse, the various types of technicians, the general practitioner, the general surgeon, the general internist and the more narrowly active specialist. Each person has made a commitment of educational time and effort to preparing for his role in the care of the ill patient. Doctors have the largest educational commitment, and society gives them the broadest license. Nurses have made a more limited commitment, and society has given them a more limited license.

Creation of New Types of Jobs to Bring New People into the Health Field

Duke University has started to produce a new worker labeled a "physician's assistant." The next few paragraphs describe that program as an example of the type of experimentation that the University believes should be going on in many medical centers.

Doctors need better assistants. They need to recruit and train colleagues who are capable of functioning in the office, in the hospital, in the laboratory or in the home and who are available, with the doctor, to meet emergency health needs around the clock. Physician assistants must have the quality of allowing irrational people (the ill) to make irrational demands on them and of meeting these demands without resentment. Physician's assistants will have to be as specialized as the doctor. They will need family at home to care for them, so that they can devote full time to the health field. They will require a salary high enough to make them not need a second job. Physician's assistants working in the health field over many years would give stability to the health-care area at the doctor-patient interface. They would keep the shop in order so that less career-minded personnel could feed in and out of the field without making the cost of retraining prohibitive.

To perform these functions one needs to recruit colleagues with good intelligence and motivation who might have been doctors if the turn of the wheel had given their families a social and financial structure to support the long general and special education needed to produce the doctor.

The belief at Duke is that persons should be selected for training as physician's assistants who have already demonstrated an aptitude and liking for work with sick people. Many bright young students with high school or junior-college training are in the medical corps of the Navy, Army, and Air Force and have the opportunity to determine their aptitude for the health area. Ambitious high-school graduates can work in a hospital and demonstrate their motivation and aptitude. It is not believed that a college degree is necessary to develop a higly trained and useful assistant. There is no wish to increase the cost of production of the assistant by too long a commitment to general education.

It will take two years to train effective assistants. In the first year they will acquire a working knowledge of anatomy, physiology, pharmacology, microbiology and electronics. They must become experienced with trauma, wound healing, suturing and handling of living tissue. In the second year the physician assistants will learn to take a history and perform a good physical examination. They will work in the recovery room, the emergency clinic, the coronary-care unit, the renal-dialysis unit and the respiratory-care unit. In the last part of the second year they can work in a private clinic, in a doctor's office, or in the admitting service of a busy hospital. If they wish to restrict their activity to one clinical area, their last few months may be spent in cardiology, allergy, pulmonary disease, renology, endocrinology or the emergency clinic.

The final duties of physician assistants must be determined by the doctor to whom they are responsible. At the time of their graduation, the medical center will record on their certificate the skills that have been developed, and will certify that they are competent to use these skills under the direction of physicians. If physicians want them to have additional skills, they can return them to the medical center for additional training and appropriate updating of their certificate. It is to be hoped that physician's assistants would not themselves be licensed, but that the schools producing them would be licensed. The responsibility for not using physician assistants beyond their degree of training would remain the responsibility of doctors.

Chapter 30

The Physician's Assistant and Internal Medicine

T he concept advanced at Duke University in 1965 that the complexities of modern practice and the need for continuing education of the doctor in practice can be effectively met by using middle-level health workers selected by doctors, educated by doctors, and paid by doctors has been proved to be correct.[1] The best recommendation for the effectiveness of the physician's assistant comes from the spouses of internists who have incorporated this new product into their practice. Doctors give more units of service per unit of time. They can care for acutely ill patients in the hospital while they are meeting their office commitments. They have protected time for relaxation, for continuing education, and for community activities.

Physician's assistants are members of the doctor's team, and their performance will mirror that of their preceptor. In theory, the physician's assistant will perform only those functions where his performance will equal that of the doctor. This requires a system of quality control, and not all doctors are equally skilled in quality control for themselves and for the physician's assistant. The doctor/physician's assistant teams show the same variations in quality that were present before the physician's assistant was

1. Stead EA, Jr. The physician's assistant and internal medicine. *Amer. J. Med.*, 70:1161-1162, 1981.

employed.

If you wish to build a complex house, you need more than lumber and glass. Copper, aluminum, steel, plastics and other materials allow you to build a more durable and energy-efficient house. To build a complex practice, you need more than the receptionist, office nurse and laboratory technician. With both hospital and office practice, you need to be in two places at the same time. The physician's assistant solves these problems of geography. *Look* magazine brought our new product to the attention of the country by a pictorial account entitled "More Than a Nurse, Less Than a Doctor."

When nurses began to get their heads above water and looked around at the post-war world, they appreciated that a new professional group was treading on turf that might have been claimed by them. Their reaction was quick and violent. Out of this frustration emerged the extension of nursing into new areas. The nurse practitioner was born.

I am frequently quizzed by nurses as to the differences between a physician's assistant and a nurse practitioner. The nurse practitioner is usually trained by other nurses and her competence is restricted by this fact. The physician's assistant is trained by doctors who have wider areas of competence than does a nurse. Physician's assistants working under the doctors can increase their competence to a level comparable to the doctor; a nurse practitioner cannot exceed the limitations of her license. Nurse practitioners commonly report to other nurses. Physician's assistants report to doctors.

There are, of course, many similarities between the nurse practitioner and the physician's assistant. I have emphasized the differences. Once in the workplace, differences from schooling may disappear. Doctors trained in a small school known only regionally may become as skilled as doctors trained in the most prestigious school with national and international reputation.

Given an effective program of continuing education, differences present at graduation may disappear. You cannot keep a good person down.

The fact that a doctor/physician's assistant team can give excellent service and that patients readily accept this team has been demonstrated in many areas of the country. A new question has arisen. Will we have more doctors than the nation can absorb? Will the income of doctors fall to a much lower level? Will we have to dismantle effective units to make more work? Will doctors need middle-class welfare?

We can accept it as a given fact that if doctors have a dramatic fall in work load and income, they will combine to kill off all nurse practitioners and all other mid-level health workers. They will attempt to revoke the license of all doctors using physician's assistants and nurse practitioners. Doctors are, after all, human and nothing brings out our humanness more quickly than a threat to our pocketbooks.

We do not know for certain that we will be over-doctored. Up to a point, our newly emerging doctors may be willing to accept a decrease in income in return for a less demanding professional life. Medical education may become a more accepted form of general education. Law has for many years been a form of general education which leads to employment in many areas besides the formal practice of law. Persons with an M.D. degree are increasingly being employed by industry and government to carry out functions unrelated to patient care. The appreciation that environmental contacts with hundreds of substances and varying physical states can produce disease has opened up new areas for employment of doctors. Ponder the number of persons now employed in premature nurseries, in testing for recessive genes, in genetic counseling, in replacing hips, and in complex cardiovascular procedures. Community-wide heart transplantation programs are just over the horizon. They await only the emergence of a holding procedure analogous to renal dialysis in the kidney transplantation program. Look at the output of basic science laboratories and the technologies that are emerging from them. List the constantly emerging specialties occurring in every major area of the health field. The economists say that we can no longer afford more health care activity. Fortunately, economics is not yet a science and their prediction may be wrong. No one 100 years ago would have believed that satellites and microprocessors would impinge on our pattern of daily living.

If work in the city slows down, the physician/physician's assistant team can easily expand into more rural areas. A physician's assistant who has worked for a time with an internist can live in a rural community. The internist/physician's assistant team can establish an office near the residence of the physician's assistant. The physician's assistant can continue to work in the urban office of the internist one or more half-days per week. The internist can work one or more days in the rural office. The supervision can be very effective if the internist has a good managerial sense. No one knows how many physician's assistants will be needed to staff offices in areas in which internists do not wish to live or in which the level of the economy would not support a full-time internist.

There are still many places where the wheel squeaks and the physician's assistant/internist team could supply the oil: prisons, reformatories, homes for mentally retarded and handicapped, geriatric nursing homes, inner city areas and rural areas. These areas represent opportunity for the physician's assistant and for internists interested in a diverse practice.

In many hospitals the physician's assistant now performs functions previously delegated to interns and residents. If working conditions are satisfactory and the physician's assistant remains a part of the doctor's team, the doctor/physician's assistant team may provide more units of service than the traditional doctor/resident/intern team. Employment by the hospital and reporting to the nursing service are less satisfactory arrangements and usually result in a higher level of turnover than is desirable.

The use of the physician's assistant on hospital services has allowed the chiefs of services to be honest. For the first time, they have the manpower and hands to cover service functions. They can now reduce the resident-intern staffs without destroying needed service activities. They can now define more precisely the number of interns and residents they need to have for educational purposes.

Chapter 31

New Roles for Personnel in Hospitals: Physician Extenders

M edical practice does not require an advanced training in science. We have a lot of bright young interns from all kinds of schools, who come to learn the science of practice and the application of science to patient care.[1] I point out that maybe it would have been just as well if they had stayed at home. I could, within a couple of days, present all the science useful in medical practice.

Now you must remember that there is a lot of knowledge in the world for many purposes, but there is so much non-knowledge when it comes to the care of patients that the proportion of non-knowledge used on any day is at least 90% of what the doctor does. Now you must appreciate that it takes some knowledge of science to make a radio. At least it takes some if there has been no radio made before. But one does not have to be a scientist to operate the radio. So the president of RCA runs his radio and I run mine, and we do it equally well. When the thing breaks down, neither of us knows what to do.

So you must differentiate between investment in science, which is related to the creation of things unknown — be it knowledge or machines or various kinds of things — and applica-

---

1. Stead EA, Jr. New roles for personnel in hospitals: Physician extenders. *Bull. N.Y. Acad. Med.*, 55:41–45, 1979.

tion of science, which in itself most of the time is relatively simple.

Along the way I have had experiences that were helpful to me in getting to where I stand now. I happened to be a professor of medicine at Emory University during World War II. We had a long negotiation about how many interns we were going to have, and it was decided that the number of interns I could have was equal to that of a date 15 years earlier. Well, at that time there were no interns, so I came up with a figure very close to zero. But I still had a lot of patients to take care of, so I calmly conscripted the third- and fourth-year students. I just said, "We've got a lot of folks to take care of: it's going to take most of the day and a fair part of the night, and I'm not asking you whether you want to do it; I'm just merely pointing out that these are the requirements and, if you stay here, this is what you're going to do and, if you don't, the Army would love to have you in another capacity."

I think the astonishing thing about it was that they gave superb medical care. You could not tell after a while the difference between the third-year student, who had never been through the last two years of medical school, and an intern. You learn by doing, and the things that a doctor does at any one moment are not terribly complex. There is a tremendous number of them so there is a lot of experience to be had. But none of the particular procedures are terribly hard.

It is only when you go to cut new paths that you require a different kind of background and a different kind of education. But I did learn that they did not need to go to medical school to learn to practice medicine. That turned out to be perfectly obvious.

My next experience came with a group of nurses at Duke University in the early 1960s. Thelma Ingles wished to train nurses to be able to give a larger quantity and variety of services.[2] So she set up a master's degree program and I agreed to interact and teach the nurses anything I knew that they wished to learn. They were very intelligent and they learned quickly, and at the end of a year we had produced a superb product, one capable of doing more than any nurse I had ever met.

Well, we fell on evil times. The nursing hierarchy would not credit that master's program. Miss Ingles went off to The Rockefeller Foundations having taught me again that people from varied backgrounds can apply knowledge very effectively at the level of patient care.

When the war ended I had more time for reflection. It became obvious that the nurses had not changed much during the period, when major changes had occurred in medical practice. I am not being critical of why they had not changed: I am merely making the statement. So the ceiling for the nurse in 1960 was approximately what it had been in 1938. And beneath that ceiling had grown a whole variety of plans: we had practical nurses; we had two-year nurses; we had diploma nurses; and we had degree nurses.

And, since bright people will learn, at the end of two or three years there was not very much difference in the performance in all those categories of nurses. Now, during that period of time, there had been a tremendous jump in the activities of doctors, so that now there was a very large gap between what the registered nurse did, what the degree nurse did, and what the doctor did. But nobody was moving into that gap.

There were technical people who took X-rays or looked at Pap smears, but nobody was moving into that gap in the area in which you actually touched people, putting hands on people — which had been the traditional role of the doctor and the nurse. And, therefore, around 1963 we elected to move into that gap

---

2. See Chapter 17, p. 107.

with a product we called "physician's assistant" and which we later changed to "physician's associate."

I had some very strong prejudices at that time and I guess it is fair to say they are still with me, but the physician's associates by and large are not included in my prejudices.

First, I am not very degree-conscious. I have always been performance-conscious. If one does something, I can appreciate it. If one gives me a degree, I do not really know what to do with it. And therefore I was interested in starting out to train people on a high-school basis.

The second thing I was interested in was the generalist. I was interested in people who could do a whole series of things. Because, when you take care of people, if you become too specialized, you tend to sit around; that special function is not needed and, you know, you smoke cigarettes or drink Coca Colas or whatever. But if you are a generalist, in the medical world there is always something to do. So I was really interested in people who were not afraid to say what the simple elements of a diet were; were not afraid to do simple portions of physiotherapy; were not afraid of taking off a bandage and putting it on; were not afraid of going into the home to see whether the older person had food in the refrigerator.

I did not see any reason people could not sew up wounds, fix simple fractures, put needles in a variety of places, or counsel individuals. You know, I wanted people just to do things. It seemed to me that the more general you made the base, the more production you could get out of the individual person.

I felt, and I still have some prejudice in that direction, that if we want to select this product, go to all the trouble to train it, eventually employ it, this could best operate as an arm of the physician and not as an arm of either the hospital or anybody else. And, indeed, this is the way my own practice goes, and my physician's associate is an extension of myself. I interact with the nursing service, the hospital administration, the nursing home administration, or what-not. The physician's assistant belongs to the medical side of this organization as contrasted with the nursing side.

Now the thing has gone very well, as you know. We suggested in 1960 that it would be better to have a managed system of care and not quite as many entrepreneurs. The establishment decided to have a tremendous increase in the entrepreneurial output and therefore we are going to have doctors running out of our ears. The question is, if you have that many entrepreneurs, how do you really manage anything? The answer may be that it just cannot be done. We made a mistake in 1960 and we have to live through it.

In all the areas in which I have seen them operate, the physician's associates have done extraordinarily well. My physician's associate has been with me 2 1/2 years and I would say she can handle almost anything; nearly anything that I know, she knows. After all, she is bright and every day she learns something.

I am at a disadvantage in a formal educational establishment. I have been teaching in medical schools since 1932, and I have still to give my first assignment; if the student stops reading, it is his responsibility, not mine. And it is amazing, if you do not have a ceiling, how many people will stick their heads higher than you ever thought they would. So I have never told anybody to stop learning.

I have always operated with a sort of open system. I appreciate that there are licensing boards, I appreciate that there are a lot of jurisdictional things, and I appreciate that there can be a lot of fears in a variety of people. My experience is that when you do not want to do something, you get very fearful. If you do want to do something, you are not nearly as fearful.

So my advice to the physician's assistants has always been to go where you are needed. Find the place where something is squeaking, and become the oil to eliminate the squeak. When you go where you are not needed and are pushing into places where people do not want you—where the shoe is not squeaking—you are much more liable to have people say: "I don't like you. It's pretty crowded here; I wish you'd get out."

So it does make sense for the physician's associates to move into areas where they actually are needed. And many of them have. Now, just one word about the relation between the physician's associates and nurse practitioners. The greatest service I ever did for nursing was to start the physician's associate program. A number of nurses began to appreciate the fact that somebody else was moving into an area which had been open a long time and which they had neglected to move into.

Therefore, I would say that the nurse-practitioner in general is a kind of child of the physician's assistant and it looks like a pretty healthy child. I have stayed with the PA program as a better prototype than the nurse-practitioner for one reason: I do not believe that people have to have ceilings put on them; I think that if you go for your training to the people who know the most, then you will have the highest ceiling. Over the years I do not know of any nurse-practitioner group that can field the faculty that the Duke physician's associate group can field. And unless that faculty becomes ceiling-minded, then the Duke-trained physician's associate will continue to be, in terms of training, more capable than the average person trained around the country.

All I can say is that now there is a considerable output of people moving into the laying on of hands, between what the nurse traditionally did up to a few years ago and what the doctor has done over these many years; and it is going to be very interesting to see how these things fall out and what roles they finally play.

I have to say regretfully that Duke University is moving

more and more toward selecting people who pass the examination easily. All faculties have always selected students with one criterion—as far as I know, only one criterion—the student who can pass the work easily and cause the faculty little trouble. Our PA course has become more formalized. It now offers a degree although it is not a requirement; we are having pharmacology and physiology taught by people who are not really concerned with giving care to patients, but who want students who will require the least time.

I think this has been an unfortunate development, but I can easily see the reason why administratively those decisions have been made.

Chapter 32

Up the Health Staircase

C an the concept of upward mobility be realistically incorporated in educational programs in the health field?[1] How
does one progress from one level of competence to a higher
level? What is the relationship between formal educational programs and on-the-job training?

We struggle with these problems at all levels. The physician's
assistant wants to be a doctor. The licensed practical nurse wants
to be a registered nurse. The inhalation therapist wants to
become a physician's assistant. The Ph.D. on the medical faculty
wishes to obtain his M.D. degree.

In the Duke Medical School, we are endeavoring to establish
the following ground rules for members of the faculty who want
an additional advanced degree:

1. A member of the faculty working toward an additional degree will not be required to conform to the
   pattern of education of the usual medical student.
2. Each year the medical school accepts an agreed-upon
   number of first-year medical students. This number
   will not be reduced when a faculty member is
   accepted into medical school.
3. Faculty members can study on their own, audit any

---

1. Stead EA, Jr. Up the health staircase. *Medical Times*, 98:213-214,
1970.

course, or be tutored by their colleagues. If they
acquire the necessary knowledge and pass an appropriate examination, he will not be required to take
the formal course or pay tuition.

4. They will pay tuition only when they are enrolled as
a full-time student.

5. Faculty members who have already shown that they
are persons of mature judgment will be allowed to
omit certain portions of the work required of the
undergraduate medical student. If, in the future, they
need the omitted material, the Medical School will
make arrangements for their instruction. This is in
line with the principle that faculty members deeply
committed to learning, and who have demonstrated
mature judgment, are not to be treated in the same
way as undergraduate medical students.

This detailed discussion demonstrates that it is hard to establish the mobility principle even at the faculty level. How much
harder it is at other levels!

The development of upward mobility among persons concerned with the delivery of personal health services has been
slow because of lack of appreciation of the fact that we are dealing with a continuum. At one end we have the family and at the
other end the most highly educated doctor. In between, there
are opportunities for many persons to take part in the delivery of
health services. The areas of responsibility assumed at any one
level are a function of the years committed to education and
training. The continuum is best shown by persons caring for the
entire person and his family. The ward attendant, the practical
nurse, the registered nurse, the degree nurse, the physician's assistant, the general practitioner, the internist, the pediatrician, the
general surgeon, the obstetrician and gynecologist all do the

same type of work. The cut-off point where each stops on the basis of his education and training is different in each case. Once one knows that the material forms a continuum, it becomes obvious that one should be able to climb from the bottom to the top. To pass from one level to the next, one should go only up. One should not have to go to the bottom each time he wants to climb another notch.

Some of the problems of upward mobility in medicine and nursing will be eased if we understand that the educational process in the area of delivery of personal health services is, indeed, a continuum. A nurse of experience who wishes to become a doctor is treated exactly as though she had had no experience in the health field. In many universities, nurses in the degree program can take electives in any area of the university except the medical school. A nurse allowed to take electives in the medical school could give more complete personal health service to her patients and would save a year's time if she should decide that she wants an M.D. degree. Once more, upward mobility is a good theoretical concept. Its implementation is very slow!

VI

Health Care and the Nation: Where Are We Going?

On May 25, 1961, President Kennedy announced that the United States would land a man safely on the moon before 1970. The resources of the nation were mobilized and the goal of moon walking was met. Many thoughtful people in this country are puzzled by the fact that we can undertake a project of this magnitude and yet have no solution for poverty, ignorance, prejudice, greed, racism and war.

Chapter 33

Family Practice

C onsumers of health services want access to practitioners of medicine who will give health maintenance services and first-line care of acute illnesses and minor trauma to all members of the family.[1] These services can be given with a small investment of the doctor's time at a low cost per unit of services. The question at issue is: can medical schools, as they presently exist in the United States, produce the doctors who will become generalists and deliver high volume, low unit cost services?

We can say that no one has yet given a clear-cut, affirmative answer to our question. The output of our medical schools continues to move toward specialization. The number of generalists taking care of families continues to decline. There is as yet no evidence that the establishment of residency programs in family medicine will reverse this trend.

The academic community is an organization dominated by specialists who contribute their expertise to the general education of students who are going to be unlike themselves and to the specialized education of students who are going to be like themselves. Their standing in the academic world results from

---

1. Stead EA, Jr. and Estes EH, 1971, *Family Practice: One View, in The Future of Medical Education*, edited by William G. Anlyan, Duke University Press, Durham, NC, p. 143, 1973. E. Harvey Estes was the Chair of Community and Family Medicine at Duke from 1966 to 1985.

their specialized knowledge which is not equally well-known to their colleagues in other fields. Family practitioners or primary physicians have to accumulate knowledge from a variety of specialists, but they have no specialized area of knowledge not known to other members of the academic community. The absence of an area of special knowledge makes it difficult to structure family medicine as a discipline within the university. We have struggled with this problem in nursing without a successful solution. Nursing has no area of expertise that is not known to other health professionals. We should not repeat in family practice programs the errors we have made in nursing. The leaders of the family practice movement appreciate their dilemma and are trying to buttress their academic standing by stressing the importance of the social sciences as a part of their educational program.

Since family practice does not have an area of specialized biomedical knowledge, the family practitioner takes additional work with specialists when he wants to increase his competence in any area of clinical medicine. This highlights what may be a fatal flaw in the residency programs for family practice. If the family practitioner goes to the specialist for additional training, why should not the student who wants to go into general practice also go to the same specialist for his graduate education? Why should not the medicine, pediatrics, obstetrics, gynecology and psychiatry taught to the family practice resident have the same quality as that taught to the specialist? Family practice programs set up outside medical centers suffer from lack of involvement of specialists in their educational programs. Family practice residency programs set up in medical centers are so artificial that they serve no real purpose. Most of their entering residents will eventually be drawn into other areas of specialization in the medical center.

Family practitioners have several characteristics that differentiate them from other doctors. They are comfortable in giving personal health services to the children, the parents and grand-parents. They accumulate knowledge about their patients through a series of short contacts over a long period of time. They are able to deliver a large number of units of health services at a low unit cost and are geographically located in a place that is easily accessible to their patients. Family practitioners extract from the total pool of knowledge the parts that are useful in delivering high volume, low unit cost health services. They perform a specialized function in the community. Because of the excellence of their performance, family practitioners are puzzled and annoyed when they are told they cannot be easily fitted into the medical school setting as faculty members.

When family practitioners are practicing medicine in the community, they are the doctor specializing in a systems engineering approach to the delivery of health care. When they are in the medical center and not engaged in family practice their unusual attributes disappear. We need to take the students to our professors of family practice and not move our family practitioners to the medical center. One solution to the problem of establishing effective family programs would be to establish family practice programs as operating arms of broadly based departments of community health sciences. Community health sciences, drawing its members from medicine, pediatrics, psychiatry, gynecology, obstetrics, business administration, systems engineering, computer science, economics, sociology and epidemiology, fits well into the present structure of universities and medical centers. Community-based professors of family practice could give this group an operating arm in the communities. A department structured in this manner could keep the medical school continually informed about the needs of the community and keep the community knowledgeable about the services available in the university.

To restate the problem: can the medical schools produce

generalists who are interested in providing high volumes, low unit cost health services to the families of the nation?. The answer for the present is probably no. What changes will have to be made to make the answer yes? The changes will have to be made (1) in the admissions policy, (2) in the curriculum in the medical schools, (3) in the faculty of the medical schools, and (4) in the graduate programs.

Changes in the Admission Policy and Curriculum of Medical Schools

Medical schools have a very restrictive admissions policy. They choose students who have received good grades in high school and college and they admit candidates from relatively few of the colleges. The object of the game is to admit students who can pass the basic science courses required in medical school. At first glance, the idea of admitting only students who are nearly certain to pass the medical school courses seems reasonable. On more careful examination it may not seem so reasonable. The necessity of passing requires that these students come from colleges with professors quite like those in the basic science years of the medical school. It imposes a rather considerable homogeneity over the entire medical profession. The professors in the colleges preparing students for medical school are primarily interested in the fact that those students whom they recommend are accepted for medical school and do well in medical school. These referring college teachers are not interested in creating heterogeneity in the medical profession. Indeed, they have no leverage to do so because their students not fitting the medical school mold would be rejected.

The basic science faculty in the medical schools are not interested in admitting students who will do family-practice. They are interested in students who will do well in their courses.

The entire intake into medicine is thus controlled by persons who will never practice medicine.

Primary medical care can be given by individual doctors who want to deliver care with their own hands or by managerial doctors who want to give primary care with a team of non-doctor helpers. Doctors delivering primary care with their own hands develop by repetition patterns of response to patients' problems that become as automatic as walking or running. They are able to give satisfactory high volume, low unit cost services with a minimum of intellectualization. They do not look on each patient as an opportunity for clinical research. They do what medicine has taught them to do and move to the next patient. They need a well-run office, good support at the technical, secretarial and nursing levels, and a place to hospitalize those patients who require a considerable investment of time. Managerial doctors delivering primary care by the team approach can develop more time for thinking and planning. They have the support of a larger organization, and they are responsible for the continued development of this organization. The team delivers health service on the basis of repetitive well-learned responses with a minimum of intellectualization. The doctor's intellectualization will be at the managerial interface rather than at the doctor-patient interface.

The medical schools need to admit three types of students: (1) the present varieties, (2) those interested in giving primary health care with their own hands, and (3) those interested in the managerial sciences. Appropriate provisions need to be made to prevent these different groups of students from being flunked out of medical school.

The students in group 2 would be selected from persons who have had experience in the delivery of personal health services and whose applications were strongly supported by practicing doctors. The students in group 3 would be those who had who had shown interest and ability in the managerial sciences and who want to become involved in the delivery of health services. Students in groups 2 and 3 would receive a four-month introductory course in the delivery of health services to allow them to function as clinical clerks. After completion of the two-year clinical clerkship, a committee of the school would decide the amounts of basic science and managerial science that the student would need to complete for the M.D. degree.

These changes would give us the necessary breadth of input to allow the schools to produce the widely differing kinds of doctors the health field needs. My own observations convince me that we could produce very effective practitioners from each of the three groups. More, but not all, of group 1 would be specialists; more but not all of group 2 would give primary care with their own hands, more but not all of group 3 would practice medicine with health teams incorporating modern methods of management. The medical center would have to develop into a working laboratory for managerial scientists not normally at home in the health field. The departments of community health sciences would need faculty knowledgeable in business administration, economics, systems engineering, bioengineering, computer science, sociology, and the epidemiology of chronic illnesses. These new faculty members would teach medical students in group 3 and interact with graduate students from their own disciplines. They would form a nucleus of those who could act at the medical center medical school interface on the one hand and at the medical school practitioner interface on the other. If successful, these new faculty members could influence medical school curriculum and admission policy and the patterns of medical care in the future.

Changes in Graduate Education

The graduate education of those students in groups 2 and 3 who want to practice Family Medicine should be under the direction of departments of community health sciences which have on their faculty physicians practicing family medicine in several communities. The Department of Community Health Sciences needs financial support for residents who can be trained in part by the traditional specialists and in part by practitioners in the community. After a year in Medicine, Obstetrics and Gynecology, Pediatrics, or Psychiatry, a Family Practice candidate can be profitably absorbed by a specialty service for the expertise the candidate brings that is not normally present on the service. A man moving from obstetrics and gynecology to medicine can function on medicine as the office gynecologist. He can work on the medical service as long as needs be at his own pace and not be a drain on the Department of Medicine budget. Since family practice will be performed in the community by single doctors and by groups of doctors, the degree of overall competence to be acquired should be left to each candidate. All required rotations tend to be dull, and uninterested rotators can kill off any service. During the period of time spent in graduate education in the medical center, the candidate for family practice should have experience in both managerial sciences and family practice in the community. The time for these experiences can be created by giving the candidate for family practice a good clinical support system. A nurse practitioner or physicians assistant would work with the family practice resident both in the medical center and in the community. Both would have access to a small computer dedicated to their system of record-keeping.

The family practitioner on the faculty would be paid for the time invested in teaching and for time devoted to effecting changes that would increase his ability to see more patients. The staff of the department of community health sciences would be a resource for the family practitioner interested in innovation.

In summary, we acknowledge the need for a more generally oriented family practitioner. We accept the fact that the production of this product requires major changes in the composition of the medical faculty, the admission and curriculum policies of the schools, and the programs of graduate education. We suggest that family practice departments staffed primarily by family practitioners will not be able to induce the changes in admissions policy, curriculum, faculty, and residency programs that must occur if generalists in large quantity are to be produced. Widely based departments of community health sciences, containing scholars capable of modifying both the medical school and the patterns of practice in the community, are more likely to succeed. This model requires that these departments have a strong operating division of family practice. The family practitioners on the faculty would remain with their practices, but they would be well paid for a portion of their time devoted to the education of students and residents.

The following paragraphs describe a proposed training program for the preparation of tomorrow's primary care physician. The program assumes that there must be a different recruit, a different training program, and a different postgraduate educational experience. It is assumed that this program will run in parallel with the conventional curriculum of a well-established medical school and be the responsibility of the Department of Community Health Sciences.

Selection of Students

Students will be chosen by a separate admissions committee who agree with the objectives of the program. Selection criteria will emphasize synthetic rather than analytic capability, interest in primary practice as a career, experience in health care and experience with geographic areas or groups in particular need of health care (rural areas, areas with a high percentage of minority residents, etc.). The students will be accepted from colleges that at present have few or no premedical students.

Preliminary Requirements

Prior to entry into the first year, the student will be asked to spend several months working in the office of a primary care physician. His role will be similar to that of a Type C physician's assistant. The purpose is to acquaint him with the type of patient seen in primary care practice and the general characteristics of the services offered, so that he will be able to contrast this with care offered in the hospital setting. For those who may have had prior health care experience, this period of time might be spent in refresher courses at the undergraduate level, if desirable.

General Characteristics of Year One

The purpose of Year 1 is to introduce students to the words commonly used by the physician and to teach them how physicians think and work. It will be spent in the medical school and its hospital. The first four months of the year are largely didactic and taught by clinicians. Studenta learn topographical anatomy and x-ray anatomy before they learn to dissect. They will meet the liver in the clinic and appreciate its function in health and disease before they meet the liver in the morbid anatomical laboratory. They will learn interviewing techniques and methods of physical and laboratory testing before they concern themselves with the sciences that have produced these methods of examination. They will learn facts about growth and development by observations of families. They will have enough epidemiology to have a grasp of the kinds of illness important in the patient population of the state. At the end of four months, they will begin their clinical clerkship. The practice of medicine is interspersed with classroom work, laboratory work and demonstrations given by select members of the basic science faculty, chosen for their ability to relate their knowledge to the problems of the patient. The clinical instructor attends the basic science exercises and relates the material presented in lectures and laboratory exercises to the problems presented by the patient.

Year Two

Year 2 will be a continuation of the clinical clerkship in that the student will be assigned to hospital wards and work under clinical preceptors. The experience will differ from the clinical year of most medical schools in that patients will be assigned to the student without regard to the nature of the admitting diagnosis. In fact, an attempt will be made to mix medical, pediatric, surgical, etc. patients in order to simulate the mix of patients likely to be seen in the primary care physician's office. The objective of the year is to teach the student to become facile in the approach to the seriously ill patient and to learn the responsibility for care of the seriously ill. Teaching rounds will be held on a daily basis, with the student and preceptor working together to derive maximal information from the attending specialist appropriate to the major problem. The base for this exercise will be in a community hospital rather than a university hospital.

Year Three

Year 3 is designed to provide some exposure to management, records, the medical system, medical planning and other components necessary for primary care practice. This material will be interspersed with patient experience in various office settings, with a large percentage of this experience being in primary practitioner clinics. The objective of the clinical experience is to provide practical knowledge of the handling of relatively minor problems, achieving rapid turnover at a reasonable cost.

This will be interdigitated with experience in relevant basic sciences such as microbiology, clinical pharmacology or pathology, and with experience in outpatient clinical settings of relevant subspecialties such as gynecology, ear-nose-throat, and dermatology.

Year Four

Year 4 of the program will be spent as a responsible clerk in a family practice program in a community hospital. The activity and responsibility will be those usually associated with an internship year. The fact that the trainee has not received the M.D. degree can be handled in one of several ways. The most interesting way is that the student could be certified as a physician's assistant and assigned to the chief of the service in the designated hospital. Thus, he would receive some benefit of legal protection under legislation now under consideration in a number of states. It is hoped that these primary practice programs will afford both inpatient experience and outpatient experience in a primary care type clinic. This clinic experience will be designed to resemble a practice setting. It should have its own record system, its own personnel, its own billing system etc. The student might also profit by receiving a small percentage of the income produced in the clinic.

Chapter 34

Why Moon Walking Is Simpler than Social Progress

On May 25, 196l, President Kennedy announced that the United States would land a man safely on the moon before 1970.[1] The resources of the nation were mobilized and the goal of moon walking was met. Many thoughtful people in this country are puzzled by the fact that we can undertake a project of this magnitude and yet have no solution for poverty, ignorance, prejudice, greed, racism and war. They declare that a country that can produce a moon stroll on schedule can solve the important social problems on this earth if it tries hard enough. They believe that our major social problems can be solved (a) by redirecting toward selected social goals the flow of funds now committed to the Vietnam war and to space exploration, and (b) by redirecting toward the solution of defined social problems the energies of the scientists and engineers now working in defense and space. Thoughtful analysis of the problem will make clear why the brilliant performances in space or defense do not lead to increased competence in preventing poverty, prejudice and pillage.

Given adequate financial support, the nation could meet its moon goal because:

---

1. Stead EA, Jr. Why moon walking is simpler than social progress. *Medical Times*, 97:248-250, 1969.

1. It was not necessary to involve all the population. One could select and choose those human beings with the necessary talents and the desire to take part in the venture.
2. The object to be built was inanimate and inanimate objects do not arouse intense feelings. Therefore, people of widely different cultures, educational backgrounds and beliefs could be mobilized to work on the space project.
3. It was possible and practical to change the design and construction of the rocket whenever the structure underway was found not to assure a functioning space ship. Any faulty part could be replaced at will. Initial errors could be corrected.

How different is the situation when man is the machine to be made! The prevention of ignorance, poverty, racism, prejudice and war depend on the accurate design and proper construction of human machines that will function to produce a society of intelligent, constructive and tolerant men. Man is made from the union of the egg and sperm. If certain elements are missing from the genetic material that programs the system, development of this human organism into an optimally-functioning person is impossible. We will forever, until the organism dies, be dealing with an imperfect instrument. We cannot replace the defective parts and construct a better design.

As the fertilized egg develops, it is highly sensitive to environmental influences which at critical times can cause permanent changes in the final machine. A drug may inhibit development of a limb bud, or rubella virus may cause minor or major defects. At birth, the nervous system is still remarkably plastic. Favorable environmental influences will favor developments useful to society; unfavorable influences will favor changes that will be detrimental to society.

In the early years, many of the changes in the nervous system produced by the interplay between hereditary and environmental influences are easily reversible. There are, however, no provisions for replacement of injured or sick nerve cells by new and viable nerve cells. The cells of the nervous system must last throughout the lifetime of the organism. The reversibility in the adult nervous system results from molecular changes within existing nerve cells, not from the addition of new cells. After the age of six, more and more of the final structure is fixed, and a smaller and smaller portion of the total structure contains reversible elements. In the early years, children can learn several languages without conscious effort. They can speak each one with the native's accent. After the age of six, the nervous system loses this ability to accept alteration from the environment without effort. Any language learned thereafter will require effort. Learning does not occur in a vacuum. Anything retained in the nervous system requires an alteration in the molecular structure of the nervous system. Any unlearning requires a change in structure. The older we become the greater must be the energy input to produce any change in structure.

The child grows and matures with his nervous system becoming more fixed each year. There is no way to redesign or replace poorly developed portions of his nervous system. Fears, hates, prejudices and poor patterns of learning and performance become permanent parts of the system. It is important to remember that prejudices and other feelings are produced by finite changes in the structure of the nervous system. They are a manifestation of molecular arrangement — not of mysticism. They cannot be altered unless one can alter nerve cells at the molecular level.

When our nation faces its social problems today, we have the problem of building a rational, cohesive society out of a series of twisted and tortured components. We have to live with what we have grown, and we have no knowledge of how to alter, to a sufficient degree to guarantee social progress, what we have grown.

It is clear that we must continue our search for knowledge for many years before we shall know how to modify the genetic and environmental factors to allow production of men who can live together in peace. Even the thought of genetic and environmental manipulations that would produce men without our present cultural characteristics and built-in prejudices frightens mankind. Peoples' feelings about people are quite different from peoples' feelings about non-human machines.

If one believes that people are free agents who can alter the structure of their nervous systems at any time by the exercise of free will, one can be optimistic about rapid social progress. If, on the other hand, one believes that adults are machines whose structures have in them a limited number of reversible elements, one must be much more pessimistic about rapid social progress. This is the answer to the question of why a nation that can send a man to the moon has no easy solution for the social problems of this earth.

As people begin to regard themselves in a more natural way, they appreciate that they are in reality machines that must operate within well-defined limits tightly bound by their structure. As they understand the growth and development of their nervous system, they will devote more energy to the health of the mothers producing the human-machines that set the limits of social progress. They will use a larger portion of their resources to affect favorably the development of human-machines during their early and more plastic years. They will pay more attention to the development of the structural changes that express themselves as feelings and lead man to destroy man.

It is important at this time that decision-makers creating

public policy understand what we must do if we wish to be able to modify man's relationship to man. Agencies designed to have an effect on social systems must be structured and programmed in an entirely different fashion from those that can produce superb engineering feats. Excellence in one area by no means assures excellence in another.

Chapter 35

A Proposal for Identification of Those Few Areas of Essential Functions that Are Not Best Served by Our Present Economic System. Can Better Systems Be Devised?

Our private enterprise system has worked reasonably well and has allowed each individual to have the privilege of arranging his own life according to his own abilities.[1] As the density of our population has increased, as the likelihood of the action of an individual hurting his neighbors has increased, as our defense needs have grown, as the number of dependent persons has risen, we have employed an increasing portion of our people in government and in government-sponsored activities. We have allowed our private enterprise system to control the rate of remuneration offered by government. When persons are drawn from government to the private sector by an increase in income in the private sector, incomes are increased in the public sector. We have agreed that in our complex society many persons will lose their ability to return a profit to their employer and that these persons will be supported by tax dollars.

We are supplying services to children, handicapped persons of all ages, to the dependent elderly, and to the military through

---

1. Stead EA, Jr. A proposal for identification of those few areas of essential functions which are not best served by our present economic system. Can better systems be devised?, unpublished essay. July 1980.

some variation of our for-profit system. By contracts with government or by direct government employment, we arrange incomes to compete with the private sector. All our systems are designed to be profitable for those engaged in them. The concept of giving services to our country because we wish to preserve it and to continue its tradition of freedom for the individual has gradually disappeared. We have embarked on a course where all service is paid for at a level that can return a profit.

We can raise the philosophical issue of whether there can be a single best way for handling all issues in a complex society. In my experience and that of others, there is never a single best way that can cover all needs. There is usually an agreed-upon best way to cover 90% of the needs but this best way is often ridiculous when applied to 10% of the problems.

I believe the time has come to examine whether this overall lesson learned from operational experience should not be applied to some major issues in our society. We can best protect our system designed for individual excellence and for profit by clearly identifying those areas where this system does not work. We need to devise alternative systems for these areas.

I suggest that the Milbank Fund appoint a panel of distinguished citizens to conduct a thoughtful examination of our present operating system, identify the problem areas that the present system cannot solve and devise alternative solutions for these problems. I will discuss four areas that I believe are insolvable by the present system.

1. *Education of children.* Enormous changes are occurring in our society. By the year 2000, a large part of our work force will be composed of the children of today, many of whom will come from the families with two working parents, from minority groups close to or below the poverty level, from households

managed by a single parent, and from welfare families. With the exception of the more affluent families where both parents work, these children must reach adulthood without the many hours of love, education and training that we are accustomed to expect from our two parents/one worker families of the past. Day nurseries and public schools are attempting to meet the needs of our children. The for-profit system has no expectation of supplying enough services to fill the void in services to our children created by our economy and by the changes in the demographic characteristics of our children.

2. *Care of dependent persons at all ages.* One can supply services at a profit to the dependent elderly from families with an above the median income. There is no humane way to make a profit out of care of all the dependent elderly. There are not enough tax dollars to support salaries of the necessary work force at a level set by the private sector.

3. *Rebuilding of our cities.* If one drives in New York City from 42nd Street to the financial district, he will appreciate that the for-profit system can never rebuild this area and at the same time care for the population now living there. One can build for the middle and upper classes but not for the entire population.

4. *Our armed forces at their present size* should not be run by the for-profit system. In a democracy, most of the people in the armed services should be there because of the fact that this is a great country and not for pay equal to that in the private sector.

I am not suggesting that implementation of this proposal be based on the acceptance of my own ideas where I think the private enterprise system has failed and will continue to fail. I do believe the time has come for careful identification of those areas, if any, that the present system will never be able to deal with in an acceptable manner.

My own suggestion for an alternative system is based on my belief that this is the greatest country in the world and offers the greatest opportunity for creative effort by each person. In return for this great gift, I believe each of us should be willing to give two years of his life, not for profit but for freedom for all the other years of his life. A universal service corps to supply identified needs not approachable by the private enterprise system is one alternative that needs serious consideration.[2]

---

2. See Chapter 44, "The Balance Between Freedom, Public and Private Enterprises and National Services," below p. 315; and Chapter 45, "A Proposal for the Creation of a Compulsory National Service Corps," below p. 321.

Chapter 36

Space Biology and Medicine—
An Unmet Challenge

The challenge to medicine and biology offered by the space age cannot be met successfully by our existing bioscientists, engineers and doctors.[1] The cost of the rocket and spaceship requires that each animal or person studied create an amount of scientifically useful data beyond that ever thought possible by our current professionals. Multiple sensors collecting data continuously from several parts of at least five systems (circulatory, respiratory, renal, neurologic and endocrine) need to be devised. The data must be collected continually over long periods of time, and the systems must be able to detect small changes accumulating over many days. The systems must have a high degree of reliability because of the high cost involved. They must operate within the constraints of weight, volume and power imposed by the space vehicle. The experimental subjects and the experimental protocols must be coordinated with a flight schedule that has in it little flexibility. No wonder the bioscientists, accustomed to working on a different animal each day and making recordings over a short time on portions of only one or more physiologic systems, are unable to devise meaningful experiments for the space vehicles. The physician and the clinical physiologist are

---

1. Stead EA, Jr. Space biology and medicine—An unmet challenge. *Medical Times*, 97:228-229, 1969.

equally unprepared for designing specific studies on man.

Space does offer the opportunity to study man and other biological systems in a new environment. One can remove the force of gravity and the effects of the day-night cycles. The confines of the space capsule allow the environment to be controlled and monitored, and offer an opportunity as yet unequalled for the study of organism-environment interactions.

NASA has appreciated that space offers opportunities for bioscience and biomedicine, but it has not appreciated the need for extensive ground-based programs to create the personnel to make the observations within the space capsules cost effective. One must develop a new ground-based cadre of scientists from many disciplines to have a meaningful approach in this area. A new mix of bioscientists, bioengineers, information scientists, biologists, physiologists, biochemists, and physicians is needed. Some institutional framework of support for them and their students must be devised.

There is no doubt that a successful bioscience and biomedical space program would pay great civilian dividends. The development of sensors capable of recording physiological data from multiple systems without breaking the skin would revolutionize the practice of medicine. The ability to measure the cumulative effects of small changes resulting from organism-environment interactions would profoundly affect the science of environmental medicine.

NASA is approaching completion of its moon-landing mission. Let us hope that in the 1970s NASA will build the ground-based competence in bioscience and biomedicine that will allow it to mount a meaningful program in space biology and medicine.

Chapter 37

A Proposal for the Creation of a Free-Standing National Academy of Medicine

M any leaders in medicine believe that there is a national need for an academy to be concerned with medicine, the health sciences, and the related health professions.[1] The field of health is so large and its problems are so urgent that a National Academy of Medicine cannot be placed under the umbrella of the National Academy of Sciences, or any other existing organi-

---

1. Proposal sent to Dr. Walsh McDermont at Cornell University Medical Center, August 14, 1969, unpublished. The cover letter for the proposal went as follows:

"Dear Walsh,

I think it will be useful if individual members of the Board of Medicine point out publicly that the methods of organization and the achievements of NASA do not help us approach the goals of achieving a better society. These approaches won't stop the Irish Catholics and the Irish Protestants from killing each other. I won't even mention the Jews and Arabs.

Enclosed is my own statement.

Sincerely,
Eugene A. Stead, Jr., MD"

In 1991, Dr. Stead wrote, "The Board of Medicine [of the National Academy] had been established by the National Academy of Science. The academy had not agreed on the creation of the Institute of Medicine and the board was hesitant about taking an independent route. My letter had some influence in getting the project off dead center."

zation, without a marked re-organization of the structure and function of the parent organization. No existing organization wants to have an active, strong Academy of Medicine because they fear that the growth of the medical section would lead to the tail wagging the dog. This document is a proposal for the creation of a free-standing National Academy of Medicine.

The Need for a National Academy of Medicine

Medicine is a learned profession deeply rooted in a number of sciences and charged with the obligation to apply them for man's benefit. Traditionally, this application is made with compassion and in accord with a widely recognized moral and ethical code. Thus the responsibilities of medicine are threefold: to generate scientific knowledge and to teach it to others; to use the knowledge for the health of an individual or a whole community; and to judge the moral and ethical propriety of each medical act that affects another human being. The activities in these three areas of responsibility require the efforts of individuals from a wide range of scientific disciplines and professions.

The rapid growth of science and technology has greatly increased the potential of medicine to meet these responsibilities. Until recently, these advances in knowledge have occurred at a pace that allowed their smooth incorporation into medical science and practice. The individual medical disciplines and specialties have been nurtured by the formation and operation of a large number of scientific or professional organizations. The extent to which these organizations have achieved their objectives has varied; however, the overall efforts, on balance, have been successful. But the rapidly accelerating pace of science and its greatly broadened impact on our society have generated forces and problems that transcend the purposes and functions of these individual scientific and professional institutions.

These advances in medical science have been attended by a rise in the expectations of our society. Yet disappointment and dissatisfaction are prevalent because of inadequacies in the delivery of personal medical services and in the solution of major problems affecting our society as a whole, e.g., the degradation of our environment. Our system for the delivery of personal medical services operates largely through the private sector of medicine. Accordingly, when the economic base for private practice has declined, as in some rural areas and central cities, the delivery system for individual medical care is weakened or withers away altogether. Such a stress in one part of the system immediately leads to serious distortions elsewhere.

Makeshift attempts have to be made to use the public health arm of the system to deliver medical care to individuals, yet this arm was not designed, and is ill-fitted, for this task. As the inadequacy of makeshifts becomes clear, more drastic remedies are proposed. Pressures arise to curtail biomedical research in the alleged interests of greater delivery without realizing that it is biomedical research that creates what there is to deliver. The educational goal of acquiring the capacity to adapt to whatever scientific or technologic innovation the future might bring is lost sight of, in movements to streamline the education to little more than the quickest way to deliver what we know now. At this point in time, there is no institution specially designed to attempt a knowledgeable reconciliation of such conflicts.

There are major ethical and moral issues related to the allocation of resources. For example, in a single university medical center, the high costs of organ transplantation, benefiting only a few patients, must be weighed against the unmet needs of a vastly greater number of other patients who conceivably could be served by that center.

Even more troublesome issues of this sort are on the horizon. A body of information is accumulating on possible effects on the growth of the nervous system (and presumably on the educability of man) of *controllable* environmental influences. These influences appear to be operative during a relatively short "critical" period late in pregnancy and in the early weeks of life. Harmful effects sustained during this relatively short period may not be wholly correctable by efforts made once the critical period is past. Here we have a situation in which the power to intervene would represent a "right" of a week-old baby. To exercise that right might run directly counter to the "right" of the parents to be free from outside interference in the raising of their child. Yet abstention from the exercise of that right on a fairly wide scale might affect an appreciable portion of the intellectual structure of our society. A more immediate issue of the same kind is created by the recently developed scientific capability to predict with accuracy that healthy couples (i.e., the "silent" carriers of the gene) have a 25% chance of having a child with cystic fibrosis, the chronic, severely invaliding disease. Preventing such pregnancies would virtually eliminate the disease from our society, but it would also entail a considerable sacrifice of individual rights. Examination of this small sample of contemporary issues reveals certain features in common. As issues, they have not arisen wholly within medicine, nor is it likely that they could be solved solely by the medical profession.

A broad range of knowledge and experience is needed, yet the problems do not appear susceptible to solution by generalists or latter-day Renaissance men. Rather, their solution would seem to require people with knowledge in depth in at least one area, but with enough breadth to be able to engage productively with experts in other fields.

By their very nature, many of the issues of the sort before us today should not be resolved by government alone, although government obviously would have to participate in their resolution. For, to a considerable extent, these issues represent matters in which the rights of the individual and the interests of society or government are in potential conflict.

Even when an issue does arise principally within a single medical sector as, for example, the issue of the proper size of the government-supported effort in basic biomedical research, an acceptable policy can no longer be formulated solely by those principally involved in that activity. To carry conviction today, it is necessary to show that a disinterested group with that mixture of knowledge and experience that permits the balancing of competing needs from a far wider constituency has been engaged in the policy determinations. But, here again, what is needed are not "social generalists," but a mixture of those deeply versed in biomedical research and those with comparable knowledge in the other fields most directly concerned.

The proper analysis of issues of such a complex and largely unprecedented character would require a considerable effort in the way of concentrated study and in the gathering of data. Such efforts and study imply the existence of an institution with a full-time scientific and professional staff as well as various groups of part-time advisers. Many leaders in medicine believe there is a national need for an academy to be concerned with medicine, the health sciences, and the related health professions.

Experience of the Board on Medicine

Three years ago, the Board on Medicine of the National Academy of Sciences was established to look at the broad issues confronting medicine and to determine if a National Academy of Medicine would be a useful device to aid in decision-making for the public and private sectors of our society. After three years, the Board is unanimously agreed that a National Academy of Medicine is needed. A proposal was made by the Board to the National Academy of Sciences to establish a National Academy of Medicine under the charter of the National Academy of Sciences. This proposal was rejected because the size and aims of the proposed Academy would require a too-great alteration in the structure of the National Academy of Sciences. The National Academy of Sciences has proposed enlargement of the present Board on Medicine. This is not a satisfactory solution to the urgent needs of medicine.

A great deal of useful information has been gained by working with the Board on Medicine. We have learned by experience that a mixed membership, with about 70% of the membership from the medical sciences and professions and about 30% from other knowledge sectors, has shown itself to be a wholly workable arrangement. The mixture of such talents has proven to be essential for proper consideration of the issues, including both those it has identified itself and those brought before it from other sources.

The work of the Board has shown the limitations imposed upon it by its small membership and lack of staff. The Board has shown itself capable of generating its own agenda for action, engaging in long-term involvement in a few major-issues, and reacting promptly to critical issues that arise suddenly. The Board has been frustrated because it has been able to concern itself with only a small portion of the issues either perceived by it or brought to it by others.

In summary, working on the Board on Medicine has highlighted the needs for a National Medical Academy. It has also shown the ineffectiveness of a small group trying to fit itself into the structure of the National Academy of Sciences.

Chapter 38

The Delivery of Health Care

E ach of us has his own notion of what actions will best help us to realize our goal of making health services available to all of our citizens.[1] One can find strong support for any of the following solutions: (1) Increase the supply of doctors by increasing the size of existing medical school classes and by creating new medical schools; (2) Recruit medical students with backgrounds different from those of our current students. (3) Train more generalists; (4) Develop the regional concept of medical care to include both preventive and therapeutic medicine; (5) Train a larger supply of nurses who nurse; (6) Upgrade the nurse to take over many of the functions of the doctor; (7) Train more women as doctors; (8) Distribute interns and residents to community hospitals; (9) Train doctors to be better managers so that they can use effectively a more complex team of assistants and thus increase their patient coverage; (10) Substitute prepayment plans for fee-for-service programs; (11) Establish a national health insurance program; (12) Enlarge the public sector of medical care to cover catastrophic illness and areas of economic and social poverty; (13) Establish corporations for the delivery of medical care as we have established corporations for the delivery of telephone service or electrical service; and (14) Pay for pre-

---

1. Stead EA, Jr. The delivery of health care. *Medical Times*, 96:216-217, 1968.

ventive care with a penalty charged to the doctor whenever his patient has to lose time because of illness.

The time has come to begin to simulate each of these solutions with appropriate models to determine which of the models are possible in terms of current manpower and resources. What would be the cost of the various models in terms of production of the needed manpower and of operation of the system? What are the professional and social constraints on the system? Are there enough nurses who want to be upgraded in professional responsibility to have an impact on health care? Are doctors good enough managers to operate larger teams? What are the constraints on the system imposed by distance? Will transportation and communication devices solve the problems of distribution?

The first models will be made with soft data in many areas. Even so they will highlight the facts that certain models are prohibitively expensive and that certain models require too many highly trained professionals. The models that seem most promising could be approached experimentally and hard data collected.

This is a country large in size and marked by great variability in population densities and economic resources. The models devised for large cities will not serve rural areas. Our nationwide health problems are not to be solved with a single answer.

Chapter 39

Unsolved Issues in Medicine:
Geriatrics as a Case in Point

A ll societies have had to solve the problems created because a minority of the people at any one time require personal services and material assistance beyond the amount that is needed by the majority of persons who are healthy and able to work.[1] Babies, children, handicapped persons, and people who become dependent because of mental problems, unemployability, or advanced age have in common the need for support systems that are more extensive than those needed by healthy adult working persons. The distinction between the dependent and independent portions of our society is clear cut when one compares a productive machinist and a baby. The distinction becomes more hazy when one considers the support system needed by single working women with one or more children and the support system needed by workers if occupational illnesses are to be prevented.

The older persons in our society present no special problems as long as they are financially solvent and can maintain the style of living that they maintained as productive members of the work force. As they lose their independence and become dependent upon other members of the society, they raise all the

---

1. Stead EA, Jr. Unsolved issues in medicine: Geriatrics as a case in point. *J. Amer. Geriatric Soc.*, 30:231-234, 1982.

issues—social, ethical, and economic—common to dependency. The geriatrician cannot, with medical skills, solve the problems of dependency, but can bring to these issues a broad perspective colored by the everyday experiences obtained by working with the elderly.

In an earlier period, many persons believed that education and improved health care combined with improved technology would reduce our dependent population to well babies, healthy children, and chronologically very old persons. They envisaged that support systems for sick and handicapped children and for persons with chronic illness, and welfare for adults unable to fit into the work force, for adults with mental disabilities, and for other disadvantaged groups, would require less and less of our resources. Unfortunately, the complexity of our society has increased at a faster pace than our ability to teach people to meet its complexity, and dependency has increased rather than decreased. "In the years 1966 to 1976 the number of persons permanently limited in their activities because of health conditions increased by 37% with a much larger proportion of those disabled claiming to be unable to carry on their main activity." During this ten-year period, our population increased by only 10%.

Many persons who can function independently in a rural family-centered society lose their independence when they have to meet the much more complex demands of an urbanized society. Medical science and technology have increased the salvage rate of fetuses and have allowed the survival but not the restoration to independence of many damaged children, accident victims, and elderly persons. In most instances, the private and public sectors still behave as if the problems of dependency will go away, and planning is done on an *ad hoc* fragmentary basis. There are no straws in the wind to indicate that progress in the biologic sciences will solve the problems of dependency. Medicine is ultimately a social as well as a biologic science.

The number of dependent persons in our society is increasing more rapidly than is the number of workers. Even if the present ratio of dependent persons to workers should remain unchanged, the dependent population would consist of many more of the elderly and fewer of the children. The demography of the work force also is changing. Welfare children of today and the children of black and Hispanic minorities will form an increasing percentage of the work force of tomorrow. In the future, we will be forced to make one or more of the following changes:

1. Increase taxation to the point where the United States becomes a completely socialistic society.
2. Work out programs by which partially dependent persons barter some services with other partially dependent groups.
3. Pay a minimum wage to every partially dependent person who can do some work. The source of the wage would be in two parts: part A paid by the person receiving the services, and part B paid by public monies to bring the income of the employed person to the level of the minimum wage.
4. Establish a national service corps and require all persons capable of working to give their services to the country for a period of two years. Payment for these years would be at the subsistence level.
5. Allow persons who are demented or likely to die within a few months to die without the intervention of modern medicine and technologically oriented support systems.

I do not believe that taxation to the point of loss of most freedoms for everyone is desirable, and I will not comment further on this alternative.

Barter services have real possibilities. Many mothers barter babysitting services. In a community of older dependent persons, exchange of services that allow persons not to be institutionalized is common. Bartering can be done without additional funds.

Bartering breaks down when one person has become so dependent as to have no services to barter. It does not work well when the income of the persons bartering the services is below the subsistence level. A possible solution is a combination of income supports that would allow a dependent person with some financial resources to purchase services at a level below the minimum wage from another less dependent person who was, in turn, supplemented by public monies to bring his income to the level of the minimum wage. The greatest obstacle to this solution is the rigidity of the federal and state bureaucracies. They have trouble in cross-linking two areas-welfare and support for the dependent-into a single system.

The establishment of a national service corps in which every person gives two years of service to the country and to fellow human beings, without expecting to be rewarded materially, is a possible solution. We have a demand for services that cannot be met by paying salaries at rates now set by the public and private sectors without increasing taxes to the point where we forego our capitalistic society. Two years of service is a small price to pay for a lifetime of freedom. The material returns to the young people in the corps would be small; the rewards of unselfish service would be large. The concept of service might well be extended beyond the two years required of the young before they become permanent members of the work force. Each of us could well give one week of service per year during our entire working life.

Our society has not faced directly the issue of allowing designated groups of persons with dementia, or with a 97% incidence of death within three months, to die without full use of support systems. We have of course faced this issue indirectly. Many persons in our country, and literally millions of persons in undeveloped countries, die each day because of lack of food, shelter, sanitation, and medical supplies. We are not interested in paying taxes to prevent these deaths. Perusal of state psychiatric institutions, state homes for children who have to be institutionalized, prisons, blighted central cities, and pockets of rural poverty indicate what we are willing to pay for, and planning is done on a fragmentary *ad hoc* basis.

Much money is spent on persons who will die within three months. As we improve our ability to determine who will die or become demented within three months, we will be under increased pressure to conserve money and accept the inevitable. I for one would rather spend the money on increasing the opportunities for children with healthy bodies and brains.

We hesitate to do by direct planning what we do by passive neglect. The ethical issues involved are many and will be avoided by the healthy workers until the material costs of not facing the issues become too high. The emergence of birth control, of new sexual freedoms, of the independent childless woman, and of the number of married couples with none to two children show that behavior can change. The society is not static.

The geriatrician caring for a dependent population must consider all the issues listed above and must give intelligent leadership to the body politic in these areas. The issues are (1) how much support to give to dependent persons and (2) how to give the agreed-on quantity of services without destroying the freedoms of the rest of society.

Once we face up to *how much*, comes the more difficult decision of to *whom*. What is due the low income, welfare, and minority mothers whose babies if properly nourished and educated will form a sizable portion of our work force? What is due the babies who appear normal? What is due the premature baby who can be kept alive by our support system, whose death a few years ago would have been certain? What is due the premature baby who can now be kept alive but only at a great risk for permanent handicaps? What is due the deformed babies, the autistic children, the children with major brain defects, those with sickle cell anemia, and those with the endless list of conditions that result in dependency? How much is due the persons who are dependent because of social conditions—disabled veterans, accident victims, victims of criminal assault, drug addicts, tobacco-induced cancer patients, the people who populate our prisons, and alcoholics? How much for the population with no education who have lived by physical labor and who are unemployable at the age of 55? How much for the dependent elderly who can live at home with some support? How much for the demented elderly who recognize no one?

The answers to the above questions reflect the belief systems of individual persons, of small and large groups, and of our society as a whole. There are those who believe the best answer is to provide maximum services and who are willing to borrow to pay for them with the assumption that our children and children's children will have new sources of wealth from which to pay back the borrowing. Others are more conservative and are more willing to set limits.

Setting limits on the dollar value of services to be supplied is difficult, but even more difficult is the decision as to the distribution of the services. Unwanted pregnancies of today produce potentially dependent persons for the next 60 to 100 years. Welfare children of today are our potential workers for tomorrow and our potential future welfare clients. Some of our dependent persons have intact brains, some are totally demented, and a number are comatose.

When financial and family resources are available to individual patients, responsible decisions on what services are meaningful and should be purchased can still be difficult. How should time and resources of the family be distributed between the demented great-grandmother, the incontinent and dependent grandmother, the working mother and father, and the children in the family? The decision is even more difficult when one must decide how much of public monies are to be spent for support of each member of the family when the mother and father are unemployed. Equal amounts of money and resources spent on each member of the family would not solve the problem. The cost of creating a personalized and clean environment for the demented great-grandmother would exceed that needed to support the young, healthy child of an alcoholic mother.

Is every unborn fetus and every person with functioning respiration and circulation to have a support system establishing an environment that would be satisfactory to the person living independently in our society? As one would expect, each of us gives a different answer when we are personally involved. Then, we want maximum support. The level of support provided to care for the severely deformed and mentally deficient children, for the mentally ill, for those on welfare, for the unemployed, for prisoners, for drug and alcohol addicts, for many disadvantaged minorities, and for the aged gives our collective answer. When we are not personally involved, we will settle for a very limited support system, and we tolerate living conditions for dependent persons that are far below the standards achieved by the independent portion of our society.

The doctor who becomes a geriatrician needs to see the broad sweep of problems that face society as it cares for dependent persons. Dollars spent on the dependent elderly are not available for education of children. When resources of a family are limited, how should they be distributed among three or four generations? Should doctors stay their hand and let pneumonia be the friend to ease the old man out of this world? If a fractured hip is repaired to relieve pain in a demented elderly person, should death from the operation be prevented by antibiotics and blood transfusions? Is it ethical for non-depressed persons facing inevitable deterioration of mental and physical facilities to arrange for their death by drugs?

While the generalization can be made that dependency in old age presents the same problem as dependency at other times of life there is at least one tangible difference: The inevitable outcome is death, and before death there will be a steady loss of function. The adult population can look at other causes of dependency and not identify with them. Old age is different. Every vigorous, active adult knows that he or she will have to die suddenly or join the dependent aged at some time. The fact of the matter is that age eventually distorts our bodies and minds, and makes us unattractive. This projection into the future creates fear in many people who are not at peace with the biologic facts of birth, reproduction, aging, and death. Combined with low pay scales, it results in a shortage of qualified persons to care for the dependent aged.

The geriatrician can help in the transition from independent living to dependency, and can frequently postpone the dependency by using every community resource to provide home care and transportation. For those who prize independence above all else, the geriatrician can persuade the family, friends, and social agencies to allow the older person to assume certain risks. Many elderly people are willing to assume the risk of a broken hip and an unattended death in order to remain independent. The old know that death is inevitable. It has happened to their friends.

Doctors have the responsibility to be certain whether the cause of the dependency is remediable. They are the gatekeepers to prevent any dependency that can be reduced or removed by scientific medicine. In a low socioeconomic group with substandard medical care, alert geriatricians will find a number of remediable medical problems. In a well-cared-for group of elderly persons of higher socioeconomic status, they will make few tenstrikes that will remove dependency.

In older persons who have decreased functional reserve in every system, acute illness can cause a rapid change in mental state, and the patient can no longer direct any aspect of his own care. Geriatricians will have talked with the family and with the older person, and they will have agreed on a course of action to be taken when acute illness occurs. Many families do not want a cardiac pacemaker to be replaced if the patient is demented. In life-threatening situations, they may not want the first pacemaker inserted if they know that the patient is existing rather than living. A decision whether antibiotics, intravenous fluids, blood transfusions, respirators, or cardiopulmonary resuscitation are to be used can usually be decided in advance of the acute problem. If the patient is admitted to a general hospital, care can be sharply directed to the acute problem and the usual routine of the hospital can be broken.

It is not an easy matter to handle the feeling states created among the nursing and attendant staff when the result is inevitable death and when the plan of care accepts death as a legitimate outcome. The amount of nursing time devoted to healing a small decubitus in a patient who is alert and responsive should be greater than the amount of nursing time spent on a large decubitus in a person so demented as to be unaware of the decubitus. The distribution of staff time is one of the areas where the geriatrician can be of real service to the nursing staff.

The family of a patient who is becoming senile and showing paranoid changes needs a great deal of help. They have to appreciate that the brain is failing and that the patient is unable to modify his behavior. The family know intellectually that the behavior, including fecal and urinary incontinence, cannot be controlled by voluntary effort, but they have a hard time integrating their intellectual knowledge into their own feeling states. As mental deterioration starts, a cycle of multiple complaints frequently begins. The patient knows that he is not well, and complaining about the body is the only way he knows to express this feeling. This type of complaining, if not understood, can cause the family and doctor to keep searching for a definitive treatable cause. None is found, and the complaining is not modified by drugs. Acceptance and understanding by family, attendants, and doctor is the only answer. An arm around the shoulder, a walk down the hall, or a glass of warm fluid is helpful.

The family, nurses, and attendants have the greatest trouble with paranoia directed toward themselves. Attendants who care for the elderly frequently come from the lowest-paid group of workers and are apt to belong to minority groups whose feelings are easily bruised. Racial slurs by the paranoid elderly patient are not uncommon. The only solution is in an understanding of behavior when the structure of the brain is deteriorating. The doctor is responsible for bringing this level of understanding to the family and attendants. The loss of independence, the fact that one's financial resources are either depleted or being depleted, and the death of close friends and associates all produce unhappiness in many elderly persons. Many doctors do not differentiate clearly between the unhappiness built into the situation and the disease called depression. In our experience, unhappiness is not drug-responsive. A human touch is the only alleviating therapy.

The question of suicide as an acceptable end for the elderly has yet to be faced by the medical profession and society. Traditionally, we are taught that taking one's own life establishes the diagnosis of depression. I do not believe this is true. Knowing the inevitability of death, one may decide on an intellectual basis that elective death is better than slow degeneration. The problems of elective dying present many hazards, and they frighten us as individuals. We wish to make the election and not have it made for us. Nevertheless, this problem will not go away. In time, mechanisms will be developed to allow the non-depressed person to have a greater role in determining the time and method of dying.

I have presented the problems facing persons who cannot support and care for themselves without special help. As long as the brain functions, each dependent person may enjoy fruitful and rewarding days. The role of the geriatrician is to see that this possibility is translated into reality for elderly persons. When medical science has nothing further to offer, good care can assure that each day is as pleasant as possible. The geriatrician wants to see the money spent where it is most effective, and recognizes the relatively minor role of scientific medicine and the more rewarding role of supplying good social, economic, and cultural support systems.

Chapter 40

Quality of Medical Care

M edicare and Medicaid are going to pump a large sum of money into the health field.[1] Theoretically one of three things might happen. First, the quality of medical care might be increased without any increase in the total amount of care rendered. Second, the present quantity of medical services might be spread over more people without an increase in the quality of services. Third, both the amount of medical care and its quality might be increased.

The first alternative is clearly out. Both Medicare and Medicaid are designed to give services to more people and an increase in quality alone is excluded by the legislation creating Medicare and Medicaid. The second alternative is clearly possible. The same quantity of total health care hours might be distributed over a larger number of people. This dilution of services — spreading the present quantity more thinly — while the money invested increases is inflation. The dollar value of the services is increased without the total services being increased. The third alternative is clearly the desirable one. More dollars should buy increased and better health services.

We will all agree that more dollars should buy increased and better health services. We will not all agree on what better

---

1. Stead EA, Jr. Quality of medical care. *Medical Times*, 95:356-359, 1967.

health services are. Each of you can appreciate the problem if you will attempt to define optimal health services in terms that apply to all individuals. My best definition is: Optimal health services are that degree of care which allows the individual to discharge his role in society with the minimal restrictions from preventable and curable illness and with the best compromises that can be made with non-preventable and non-changeable illnesses. This definition at least emphasizes the problem. What is optimal health care for one is not optimal health care for another. Optimal health care must be individualized.

We can agree reasonably well on what is optimal care for infants, children and pregnant women. We know what can be done to prevent known illness, we know the food requirements for growth and development and we know how to give prenatal care. We know that many of our infants, children and pregnant women do not receive optimal medical care. We can demonstrate this by the statistics on infant and child mortality or we can document it by the number of instances in which medical records show that the patient received much less than optimal care. It is clear that more medical care alone will not solve the problems of poverty, poor housing, slothfulness, illiteracy, drunkenness and lack of a family structure. Nevertheless we can agree on standards of optimal care for the infants, the children and the mothers, and we can document whether or not this care was given.

In the adult group we have more difficulty both in defining medical care and in determining what medical and nonmedical factors prevent the individual from receiving optimal medical care. Any obese person, smoking cigarettes and driving his car away from a cocktail party is clearly receiving less than optimal health care. He may well have been offered good services but he has clearly declined them.

Health services to adults can be divided into four general areas. (1) Relief of symptoms that are troublesome to the patient.

(2) Prevention of diseases that have not yet appeared. (3) Treatment of illnesses that are detectable by appropriate examinations but are asymptomatic. (4) Demonstration of health—or lack of it—so that persons with disease will not be given assignments that endanger others (for example, airplane pilots) and so that certain groups can be insured cheaply.

The quality of health care in the first group can be monitored (a) by the result and (b) by the record. It is hard to argue with the effectiveness of the care if the patient loses his symptoms. We know that in many instances, the recovery was not related to the diagnostic and therapeutic procedures. But who cares?

If the symptoms persist, monitoring of the record will determine whether accepted methods of diagnosis and treatment were employed. What about the cost? Here the matter becomes more sticky. What is the cost of an omitted procedure that might have changed the approach to the problem? What parts of the examination and testing could have been safely omitted? One doctor collects the needed information and makes his decision in half the time of another doctor. One doctor relies on the judgment of another doctor. One doctor rechecks a problem as if physicians seen earlier had done nothing. What is such a recheck worth? It is clearly worth more if something was overlooked or if the situation has changed. It is wasted time and money if no new information is obtained. Alas! There are no sharp answers to these problems.

The second phase of adult health care-prevention of diseases that have not yet appeared—is still in its infancy. As we identify unfavorable heterozygotes, genetic counseling will come into its own. The identification of genetic markers, which will tell us that disease may rear its ugly head in the present generation if the environment is not properly controlled, is just beginning. Primaquine sensitivity is a good example of the type of problem that will confront the doctor as our knowledge of human biology grows. Optimal health care in these areas requires both an increase in knowledge and an improvement in our methods of getting the individual to use the knowledge we have. Again optimal health care has to be defined by the ability of the individual to receive it. Wasted health care is, in no sense, optimal.

Area three, evaluation of the quality of care in persons with diseases now present but not symptomatic, is particularly difficult. All such diagnostic and therapeutic measures involve use of health personnel and require an investment of both time and money by the patient. Many people who consider themselves well do not have the reserve emotional strength and financial resources to invest heavily in preventive medicine. This is even more true when the fit between the organism and the environment is such that it causes symptoms. The person who has decompensated because of poor use of his body under the multiple stresses of our society frequently goes to the doctor for help. In this setting early diabetes, mild hypertension or obesity is likely to be found. Attempts to prevent more disease in the future by loading the situation with time-demanding and expensive medical care may result in more decompensation. What in one setting is optimal medical care may in another be disastrous. Identification of early disease, the treatment of which requires patient cooperation, is not profitable in that segment of society immobilized by poverty and illiteracy. Again optimal care must be defined in terms of the patient receiving it.

Finally, there are certain situations in which optimal medical care requires the use of particular procedures because of the occupation of the patient. Sudden death or hemiplegia in an airplane pilot may kill a hundred persons. Optimal health care of pilots cannot, in good judgment, be equated with optimal health care for school teachers, for instance.

The records of the public services of our teaching hospitals are not very useful in establishing a baseline for optimal health care overall. The teaching hospitals are concerned primarily with the conversion of raw manpower into skilled manpower for use in the health professions. The records that are kept, the diagnostic procedures that are ordered and the treatments that are administered are designed primarily to meet the needs of manpower production. The impact of such health services on the individual patient who is functioning poorly in our society is not great because cultural, economic and social and educational deficiencies prevent the operation at home of the schedules carefully worked out in the hospital. The usefulness of the doctor to society is shown more easily in those teaching hospitals that care for private patients. The medical records, the diagnostic tests and the therapeutic procedures necessary to train manpower to care for *all* patients, poor and rich, illiterate and literate, young and old, are not useful in determining what should be done to assure optimal medical care for a given *individual*. If the differences between manpower converting systems and the giving of medical care by trained manpower are not clearly appreciated, medical care will become unduly expensive and quality will not be improved.

Determining the quality of health care is a most complex problem and we need new and better methods. For the present we must emphasize the complexity of the problem and be certain that unrealistic and unworkable criteria to measure the quality of medical care are not accepted.

Chapter 41

"Clinical Trials" for Proposed Legislation?

M edicaid is a striking example of the passage of a law without adequate information being available to the Congress or Executive[1]. In the absence of a uniform federal-state system of data gathering, there was no possible way to estimate the actual impact and cost of this legislation on health care. This legislation was proposed and passed by the Congress. They had to pass it or not pass it. No mechanism existed to field-test in advance any of the component parts.

There are already a great many laws affecting the health field and each year there will be more. Doctors out in the field are aware of the problems created by these laws and by the operating agencies produced by them. Once the laws are put into operation, they gain support at the agency level. The new agencies, and the personnel employed by them, become part of the large governmental bureaucracy. Regardless of the absurdities that develop, or the lack of progress in achieving the goals that the lawmakers envisaged, the new agencies will not disappear.

Anyone who has tried to develop a sensible building program in a medical center involving facilities for education, ambulatory patients, bed patients, animals, research, library and the community becomes aware of the fragmentation of health

---

1. Stead EA, Jr. "Clinical trials" for proposed legislation? *Medical Times*, 97:187-188.

funds among governmental agencies and the inability of any one area in government to coordinate all the many avenues for support to achieve the overall objectives for which the lawmakers think they passed the laws. Even more discouragement will occur if one attempts to instigate new programs which involve a marriage between agencies supporting welfare, vocational training, education, new careers and health care for the disabled and the aged. You will find many statements of good will but no real help.

The time has come for the Congress to address itself to ways and means of testing legislation by appropriate studies before it enacts legislation that will have an unpredictable effect on our nation. We need a program of research to study the mechanisms for constructing laws that will more nearly achieve the goals for which they were designed.

My suggestion would be to make funds available to the major committees of the Congress for initiation of pilot projects before passing legislation that will affect the entire country. The laws as now passed frequently allow for demonstration projects under the new public laws. The law is so constructed that the demonstration project operates within very narrow confines, because the overlapping and functionally-related areas were not identified in the legislation. A demonstration project before the passage of final legislation would seem to be a better approach.

Further study may show that my proposal for approaching this difficult problem is unwise and that there is a better way to solve the problem. The proposal is not made to defend but rather as a means of drawing attention to the serious need for research and experimentation to improve mechanisms for designing legislation.

Chapter 42

Cost Conscious Doctors

Volume II of the Report of the *National Advisory Commission on Health Manpower* has just crossed my desk.[1] This volume is a series of appendices which gives much of the source material from which Volume I of the report was derived. The description of the *Kaiser Foundation Medical Care Program* was of particular interest to me.

The Kaiser Foundation Health Plan enrolls the patients, contracts with its hospitals and clinics for facilities to give inpatient and outpatient care, and contracts with independent partnerships or associations of physicians for professional services. The Kaiser Foundation Health Plan has the same board of directors as the Kaiser Foundation Hospitals. The directors of the Health Plan and of the Kaiser Foundation Hospitals review the proposed annual budgets of the hospitals. The hospitals do not formulate policy or expand at an independent rate.

Professional services are provided to subscribers by four Medical Groups, one in each geographic area. Organized as independent partnerships or associations of physicians, the Groups contract with the Health Plan to provide health services at a fixed charge per subscriber. Each Medical Group is autonomous and free to negotiate its own contract with the

---

1. Stead EA, Jr. Cost conscious doctors. *Medical Times*, 96:947-948. 1968.

Health Plan. For each region, a Medical Group takes responsibility for both the availability and the quality of the medical care. Patients are free to choose any physician within the Group and to change physicians at any time. As is common in solo practice, a patient may be delayed in seeing his personal physician, but immediate service may be obtained from the physician on call. This program provides comprehensive health care services to over 1.5 million subscribers on a prepaid basis. The consumer makes his wishes known through the dual choice that Kaiser has insisted be available to any subscriber. Thus, periodically any individual subscriber can choose to withdraw from the Plan and enroll in Blue Cross/Blue Shield or commercial insurance or any other system of his choice. Many do change each year, but on balance the flow has been from other plans into Kaiser.

The Health Plan has devised a system where both the doctors and the hospital profit if costs are held below the levels budgeted. These savings are reflected on the one hand in an increased income to the doctor and on the other in increased money for expansion of the hospital system. This incentive system where both professional and managerial partners have a direct economic stake in the successful and efficient operation of the overall program has resulted in significant savings to the consumer by comparison with the cost for equivalent services purchased in the surrounding communities and the country at large. The Kaiser physicians operate in a setting that makes them constantly aware of the costs associated with providing medical services and that exerts pressure on them to avoid waste. The economies effected by the Health Plan are primarily due to a decrease in hospital admissions.

I have described the Kaiser Plan in some detail because most systems of medical practice do not have a reward for efficiency built into them. At Duke the practice of medicine is carried out by members of the staff who have organized themselves into two diagnostic clinics. These clinics are directed by the physicians and all overhead charges come from their fees. If the overhead of the clinic goes up, the doctors' income goes down. The individual doctors are interested in the management of the clinics. These doctors care for their patients in Duke Hospital. Their income is not altered by achieving efficiency in the use of the hospital. Their interest in efficient use of the hospital is less than their interest in the efficient use of the clinic. The fact that doctors respond to appropriate incentive systems doesn't mean that we are mean and nasty people. It does mean that we are human!

Chapter 43

The Duke Plan

How to give public assistance with dignity; how to share the cost of public assistance between the private and public sectors of our society; how to create useful jobs for that portion of society who can work but who, if paid the minimum wage, cannot return a profit to their employer; how to give home services to the rich and poor of all races in times of need so they can live in security outside of nursing homes; how to create for the unskilled career ladders that have sufficiently small steps to be realistic; how to prevent the recycling of dependency by appropriate attention to the young; how to build a home support system that will allow professionally trained women to work and maintain their homes. These are some of the burning questions of our time. The Duke University Medical Center is developing a program that will give new answers to these difficult problems.

The Duke plan accepts the fact that public assistance will always be a necessary component of our society.[1] Indeed, we anticipate that more, and not fewer, persons will need public assistance in the future. Each person must reach a certain level of adaptability, of education and of skills to survive in our

---

1. Stead EA, Jr. 1969. The Duke Plan, unpublished as such. However parts of this essay were published as an essay, "Public assistance and society." *Medical Times*, 97:231-232, 1969. This proposal was never implemented by Duke administrators.

society without public assistance. The level that must be attained in order to maintain independence is rising at a more rapid rate than the abilities of our people. We do not believe that the people requiring public assistance need to belong to any one segment of our society, and we do not believe that children of persons receiving public assistance should automatically be the persons receiving public assistance when they reach adulthood. Instead, we look on public assistance as a necessary support mechanism which may in one generation be needed by anyone in our society. Out of the pool of persons supported by public assistance in any one generation should emerge many independent citizens of the next generation.

Those who believe that public assistance is undesirable and that recipients of public assistance are unworthy persons have always structured the system as a pure welfare program. Those of us who believe that the growth of our society demands that public assistance be available and be non-degrading wish to construct the system using funds from both the public and private sectors of our society. We believe that private agencies supported by both public and private funds offer many advantages over the present welfare system.

There are many workers who are only just able to survive on the income they create and who will eventually turn toward public assistance as they grow older. These persons receive less than the minimum wage and are not able to raise their children in a way that will make the children useful citizens for tomorrow. They have the option of continuing to struggle to support themselves or of falling back on welfare. Illness or aging may remove the option and make welfare the only recourse. In this segment of our society, we need to combine public and private moneys to provide minimal wages and to support training to increase the income potential.

The health field is the best area in our society to create jobs that can give real satisfaction to the worker who is limited in education or work skills. The children, the handicapped, the ill and the aged all require help whether they remain in their homes or whether they are placed in institutions. Anyone who can establish regular work habits can perform a useful service. At one end of the spectrum we have people of limited skills who need work and, at the other, we have the sick, the handicapped, the children and the aged who need help. The unskilled persons need a minimal wage to function in our society, and the people needing the help frequently cannot pay that much for the services. Both the unskilled worker and those needing help are frequently forced entirely back onto public assistance. A mechanism should be found by which the unskilled worker can work with dignity, and the sick and aged can receive his services.

The unskilled person entering the work force should have the opportunity to learn and to improve his condition. Many people can do this if the steps in the career ladder are small and if the entire program is geared to allow the person to make use of the material he has learned.

There are many trained professional women who work for only a few years in the health field. They are attractive and capable, and they acquire husbands. They do not need to work for economic reasons, and they have difficulty in obtaining help in their homes that would free them for services outside the home. Day care centers do not solve their problems. They need help in the home with housekeeping, budgeting, dietetics, shopping and cooking.

These trained professional workers represent an unused resource. They could work outside the home to give needed services in the health field, or they could serve as trainers of unskilled persons by using their home as the school.

Under the Duke plan the Duke Medical Center will employ, at the minimal wage rate, men and women who are now on relief or who are employed at less than the minimal wage. There will be no means test. The only requirements are the ability to establish regular working hours and the absence of destructive patterns of behavior. After a short period in service training, the services of this corps of workers will be offered as a fringe benefit to professional women working in the University and Medical Center, or to professional women now in the home who would like to return to work.

The professional woman will work from one to five days in the University or Medical Center and will spend one day per week giving instruction in the home to the home worker. She will be supplied with instruction kits, covering the areas of cooking, nutrition, shopping, budgeting, dietetics, housecleaning, care of pregnant women, bottle and breast feeding, first aid, simple physiotherapy for persons with arthritis and strokes, and nursing care for bedridden persons. Special arrangements will have to be made for those who cannot read or write. Standardized tests will be given to determine whether the training in the home compares with that given in the classroom.

The Medical Center will determine the economic value of the services rendered in the home, and this will be deducted from the pay of the professional woman. If she accepts the fringe benefit in lieu of salary, there will be some income tax advantages to the professional woman. She will also receive some income tax relief by using her home as a training base. The Medical Center will collect from public assistance the difference between the value of the services rendered and the minimum wage.

Some persons will never advance beyond this first stage of home worker. They may never create a minimum wage. They will continue to be subsidized by public assistance, but neither the worker nor the person receiving the fringe benefit of home services will know that public assistance is paying part of the bill. Some of the home workers will create a minimal wage from the start and will need no direct help from public assistance. The workers who have learned new skills from the home instructional program will be brought from the home into the healthcare institutions where they can function as aides in nursing, dietetics, physiotherapy, housekeeping, laboratory work and dentistry.

Those persons capable of advancing further in the health field will be given practical nursing training. The Duke Medical Center will maintain records of the home training and the in-service training so that due credit can be given for past achievements. Practical nurses who wish to develop further will be trained as clinical specialists, which will give them clinical skills in specialized areas equal to those of the registered nurse.

The Duke plan can be used for both men and women but, in the beginning, it will involve more women, and these women have children. Day care centers are an integral part of the program if we wish to interrupt the dependency cycle. Development in this area again needs a proper balance between public and private funding.

With this new cadre of workers the Duke Medical Center will supply home services to handicapped, ill, or aged persons who at present have to be institutionalized because they have no other resources. All persons, black or white, young or old, rich or poor at times need the help of other human beings. We wish to establish a human resource to meet the need. The Duke Medical Center will supply the persons to give the service. Duke will collect from the person receiving the services—whatever he is able to pay. Duke will bill public assistance for the difference between that figure and the cost of the services. The worker giving the services and the patient receiving the services will not know whether or not funds from public assistance are being used. Under the Duke plan the land will still be largely covered by 8-lane highways but the spaces between will not have to be filled with concrete-block nursing homes.

The Duke Medical Center believes that this proposal warrants serious attention. It has aroused interest in everyone who has seen it. The plan will be difficult to implement at the usual agency level within the Department of Health, Education and Welfare. It involves use of welfare funds; it creates new jobs in the health field; it starts a series of home schools that require central record room keeping; it needs a day care center.

Chapter 44

The Balance Between Freedom, Public and Private Enterprises and National Service

O ur private enterprise system has worked reasonably well and has allowed each individual to have the privilege of arranging his own life according to his own abilities.[1] Intuition and experience have taught us that there is usually an agreed upon best way to solve about 90% of problems involving people but that this best way does not make sense when applied to 100% of problems. Granting that the productivity and freedoms given by the private enterprise for-profit system have worked well for the majority of problems of our society, can they be the answer for a minority of problems that may eat away at our society and destroy what we all hold dear?

I believe that we can identify a series of crucial problems that will not be solved by our "for profit" system and will not be solved by the public sector under our currently accepted policies. Before identifying a series of problems with no solutions in either the private or the public sector, we should consider why the traditional policy of asking the public sector to solve the problems not solvable by the private sector no longer works.

For many years the public sector has provided services that were too expensive for the family or the individual to finance.

1. Stead EA, Jr. The Balance Between Freedom, Public and Private Enterprises and National Services, unpublished essay. September 22, 1980.

Care of persons with tuberculosis and mental illness was largely financed from tax-derived dollars. The costs of building roads, airports, hospitals and defending our country have been joint enterprises involving the public and private sectors. In general, the philosophy was that tax-funded enterprises served the common good and that they could be funded at a level of tax that did not destroy the private sector.

Until recent years a large part of the services required to operate the nation have been given at a level of pay below that of the private sector. Public service in the municipal, state and federal establishments was priced at a relatively low level. The work performed by women in homes was not recognized in paychecks and women in industry were paid wages far below those of men. There was no minimum wage. The unskilled, unemployable persons were hired by municipal institutions. Until recently, employment in hospitals was viewed as part of the welfare system. Public institutions could meet their responsibilities at a workable level of taxation and the public debt could be kept at responsible levels.

In recent years the relations between public and private sectors have changed. The income level of workers in the public sector is increasingly pegged to the private sector. Assuming for a moment that the public and private sectors can perform a function equally well, there is little cost differential. If the public sector is less efficient, a large cost differential rapidly develops in favor of the private sector. The proportion of persons working for the government or supported by welfare, Social Security, Medicare and Medicaid, and government pensions has increased dramatically. The proportion of productive persons creating the funds to be taxed is decreasing and as our population ages this trend will be accelerated. Mature societies in the Scandinavian countries have tried to solve their problems by increasing protection by government activities that. are funded by ever higher taxes. It appears that they have largely destroyed their private enterprise systems and are left with a large number of unsolved problems. Better answers are needed than more government and more taxes.

We should develop the belief in our people that our country and private enterprise system are worth saving and that this requires each of us to give services to our country that are priced far below the "for-profit" level. Universal service for each man and woman could be the unifying bond to bring our people closer and allow them to share a common experience. The manpower to tackle a list of presently unsolvable problems would be available. Two years of service for a lifetime of freedom is a good bargain. Many persons would elect to continue giving seven to 28 days of service annually to the country. Many of the gaps in the culture that are produced by age differences could be closed,

The time has come to establish an ongoing panel of distinguished citizens from all sectors of society to determine if there are critical problems threatening our way of life that cannot be solved by the public and private sectors operating under current ground rules. If my analysis is correct and such problems exist, they should be identified and alternative strategies developed. The alternative strategies would require changes in attitudes and perceptions that cannot occur quickly. Television and print consistently and purposefully used can induce attitudinal changes when they are employed effectively over years. A committee report in itself would produce no change. We would need a sustained effort comparable to that initiated by John Gardner when he developed "Common Cause."

My own interest in identifying potentially destructive situations and developing alternative solutions lies in my belief that this is the greatest country in the world and offers the greatest opportunity for creative effort by each person. The stakes are high, the chances for success not great, but a successful venture would pay immeasurable returns.

The freedom to fail in a good cause is one of the freedoms that have made our country great. Great successes are accomplished by dedicated persons who strive for success but are not destroyed by the possibility of failure. I hope that the Milbank Fund and the Commonwealth Foundation will assemble a small group of concerned persons to discuss the ideas expressed in this paper.

Chapter 45

A Proposal for the Creation of a Compulsory National Service Corps

U nited States citizens are fouling their nest.[1] We are producing more people than we can educate, house, transport, and nourish. We are supplying an abundance of material things to two-thirds of our people, but, in transforming our natural resources into electricity, gasoline engines, nuclear power, paper, beer cans, bottles, broken-down cars, rusting ships, polluted water, noxious gases, human feces, and other forms of garbage, we are destroying the environment that allows us to exist and gives dignity and satisfaction to our living.

The problem of pollution exists everywhere and threatens alike the rich and the poor. Eventually, this threat to existence will cause the establishment to move. Steps will be taken to make appropriate changes for the use of natural resources, and the producers of cans, bottles, and effluents will have to include the price of disposal as a part of the production cost. Ways will be found to recycle our waste products back into the production cycle. These changes will be difficult, but our present form of society and our present government can eventually deal with them.

All of our citizens are threatened by the pollution of our air, land, and water. The saving of our environment will solve many

---

1. Stead EA, Jr. A proposal for the creation of a compulsory National Service Corps. *Arch. Intern Med.* 127:89-90, 1971.

of the problems of four fifths of our citizens, but one fifth of our citizens will still live in poverty. This one fifth requires tremendous investments in housing, education, medical care, nutrition, and transportation. The rate of growth of this population exceeds the ability of our society to supply these people with the essentials of modern-day living. One has only to ride through the poverty-stricken areas of New York, Baltimore, Philadelphia, or Washington, D.C., to appreciate the magnitude of the problem.

We cannot possibly educate the children, build the housing, supply the transportation systems, give the medical care, improve the nutrition, and supply needed income to our disadvantaged people with the expectation of making a profit. No profit-oriented business can stand these expenses over the long period of time needed and still survive. Profits may be made in future generations, but they will certainly not be made in this one.

When private enterprise and the profit motive have not supported projects that are essential to society, we have in the past turned to support by taxation. When hospitalization of the mentally ill and of patients with tuberculosis could not be accomplished by our private enterprise system, support of these functions was taken over by government. Why cannot government collect enough money by taxation to solve the problems of our poor? The first and simplest reason is the magnitude of the problem. The rate of population growth of the disadvantaged and their concentration in urban ghettos has created a problem of greater magnitude than our government has ever had to solve. The proportion of our income that will have to go into taxes to solve the health, education, and housing problems of this one fifth of our population exceeds in magnitude any program the federal, state, and local governments have ever undertaken.

The second and more important reason why we cannot levy the taxes necessary to meet the income needs of the lower one fifth of our society is the feeling, on the part of our people who have achieved enough income to pay for the education, health care, housing, food, and transportation for their families, that they themselves are worthy and that those who have not made it are unworthy. Nothing irks the worthy more than to have to give of their resources to help the unworthy. The persons between 35 and 65 who control the wealth of this country will simply refuse to tax themselves to the point where they can solve the problems of the relatively helpless one fifth of our people. They will be taxed for wars, defense, transportation, space exploration, cities under the sea, and for a wide variety of material things. They will not be taxed to support the unworthy. The worthy are unwilling to be taxed to support the unworthy because the worthy are not good biologists. They still believe that human behavior is a mystical function and that the unworthy could be worthy if they only would. They do not appreciate that human behavior is a manifestation of the organization of the nervous system and that the structure of the nervous system at any one moment determines the behavior of the organism at that moment. A combination of genetic and environmental factors fashions our nervous systems into a biological machine. The cycling and performance of those machines determines our behavior and, in the eyes of our neighbors, our social worth. One can destroy a small part of the brain of the most worthy man and convert him into a person worthless to society. I have never given any personal credit to people who best serve the society. Their behavior reflects the organization of their nervous system, and they cannot help but be effective. I have never blamed those persons who do not serve the society well. Unless their nervous systems can be changed, they cannot become more effective. We have to live with the people we have reared. Many of them cannot go it alone and will need help over their lifetime. This false belief that the worthy succeed by their own efforts and the unworthy fail because of lack of their own efforts is too deeply ingrained into our society to combat in the space of a few generations. If we wish to help the disadvantaged in the next 100 years, we must think up some nonprofit-oriented way that is not based entirely on taxation. The worthy, in their middle years, are much more willing to give the services of their children than to give their dollars. Giving service to the unworthy has always been accepted in our society.

William Anlyan, M.D., vice-president of Duke University, has emphasized that the health needs of the nation can be met only by asking each doctor to give two years of his life to some form of national health service. I believe he is correct. When this move is made, our young doctors will discover that health and medical care cannot be satisfactorily given without solving the problems of housing, education, transportation, nutrition, and pollution. These problems can be tackled if every young man and every young woman in our country gives two years of service to the society. We need a national service corps—not just a national health corps.

I am aware that Hitler used a national service corps to prepare for war. Any device can be put to poor use. The American Service Corps can be used to prepare for living.

As the density of our population and the complexity of our society increase, each person has to make a greater contribution to the society and each must give up some of his freedom as an individual. The need for personal health services for all of our citizens is sufficiently acute to require this change in our way of living. A community with so few cars that no traffic lights are needed is, in some ways, blest. If that community grows larger and still refuses regulation of its traffic, chaos occurs. Many thoughtful people believe that the time has come when our society must ask of its health professionals these two years of service in order to avoid chaos. Giving up two years of freedom to work for society at large will preserve many more degrees of freedom over the remainder of one's professional life.

The deployment of our young, idealistic and capable professionals into ghettos, into rural areas, onto Indian reservations, into prisons, into our state institutions, will bring an inevitable reaction. The health professionals will find that ignorance, filth, poverty, prejudices, inadequate housing, poor transportation, lack of job opportunity, malnutrition and crime prevent the improvement of health, and that the best efforts of doctors, nurses and their teams come to naught. They will begin to appreciate the hard fact that to solve the urgent problems of our society *all* persons will have to give two years of their best effort to society. Eventually we will have to implement not just a National Health Service but a National Service Corps with a broader base in which each young man and young woman give two years to the society in return for the freedoms the society can offer them over the rest of their life.

There are two alternatives to a universal service corps with restriction of freedom of choice for a limited period of time. We can change our political institutions so that we accept close regulation of our lives at all times. Communist and fascist models are available. The second alternative is to attempt to accomplish the tremendous changes needed by taxation. The ethos of our society is strongly against the necessary taxes. We would be taking money from our more wealthy and successful middle-aged citizens (in their own eyes, the worthy citizens) and giving the fruits of their labor to the nonsuccessful (in the eyes of the taxpayer, the unworthy). The worthy have strong feelings about giving of their goods to the unworthy. However, in the missionary tradition, they have much less objection to giving the services of their young in the cause of people who have not made it on their own in our society.

A universal service corps could be the new melting pot of America. If all groups share in the venture, all would move from their own neighborhoods to other neighborhoods. The problem of segregation would disappear for the duration of one's time in the National Service Corps.

Chapter 46

The Opportunities for a Research Program on Myocardial Infarction: The Report of the National Heart Institute Ad Hoc Committee

T his committee came into existence because of certain convictions of Dr. Robert P. Grant, the late Director of the National Heart Institute.[1] He believed that coronary arterial disease and myocardial infarction were the greatest killers of American citizens in their productive prime, and that the resources of the scientific community were not adequately mobilized to reduce the mortality of these illnesses. He noted that although an artificial heart would eventually be made workable, the knowledge did not exist which would allow the proper identification of those persons with coronary disease who could best profit by this device. More importantly, he believed that research might provide means for salvaging a larger part of the population at risk

---

1. The Opportunities for a Research Program on Myocardial Infarction: The Report of the National Heart Institute Ad Hoc Committee. Eugene A. Stead, Jr., was chair of this committee of the National Heart Institute in 1966. Also on the committee were Drs. Richard L. Varco, James V. Warren, and Peter L. Frommer. The outcome of this committee, the formation of the National Heart Institute Myocardial Infarction Research Units (MIRUs), changed the care of patients with myocardial infarction in the United States.

and reduce the number of patients who might become candidates for an artificial heart.

The necessity for an expanded research program in the medical management of acute myocardial infarction as an integral portion of the Artificial Heart—Myocardial Infarction Program has been accepted by the National Heart Institute and the Public Health Service. In anticipation of this, this committee was appointed by Dr. Grant to survey research efforts in areas relevant to the treatment of acute myocardial infarction and to make recommendations as to how research support might catalyze activity aimed at a better understanding of this disease, with a reduction in mortality as its ultimate goal.

To develop a basis for these recommendations, 20 visits were made to cardiovascular research institutions in the United States and Great Britain.[2] The committee sought to learn the current activities and future research plans of these units. We sought to identify the constraints upon clinical research on myocardial infarction: practical, ethical and logistic—including also problems of facilities, personnel, funding and administration. Most importantly, we sought to assess the scope of new ideas for attacking the problems of myocardial infarction, and the potential commitment of scientists to the goals of this program.

In the course of our visits, we discussed a series of topics

---

2. University of Chicago, University of Minnesota, New York Hospital, Maimonides Hospital (Brooklyn), New York University Medical Center, State University of New York (Brooklyn), Postgraduate Medical School (London), Radcliff Infirmary (Oxford), Royal Infirmary (Edinburgh), Cox Coronary Heart Institute, Ohio State University, Cincinnati Veterans Administration Hospital, Jewish Hospital (Cincinnati), Tulane University, University of Alabama, Emory University, University of Southern California, Cedars-Sinai Medical Center, Baylor University, Johns Hopkins University, Peter Bent Brigham Hospital.

with our colleagues in an effort to define the research potential of a program directed at the improvement of the therapy of acute myocardial infarction. The results of these discussions and the reaction of the committee to a number of problems are summarized under the series of topic headings listed in the outline of this report.

The Pathophysiology of Infarction

The traditional concepts of myocardial infarction are undergoing change. There is general agreement that coronary atherosclerosis is intimately and almost always necessarily involved in the process, and there is the increasing realization that the conventional explanation of thrombosis precipitating infarction is not adequate. Numerous pathologic studies have demonstrated that only a relatively small portion of hearts with acute myocardial infarction have evidence of an acute thrombosis. There has even been some suggestion that thrombosis may follow infarction, rather than precede it. Just why cell death and infarction occur is not known. There is little research activity specifically aimed at understanding the pathologic processes that lead to infarction. There are a limited number of investigations measuring chemical factors such as lactate production as an indirect means of measuring cellular activity. Only a few laboratories are engaged in achieving more accurate microscopy and histochemistry of the myocardial cells as they are involved in ischemia and infarction. It would appear to the committee that the nature of myocardial infarction remains a problem of major importance that is currently receiving relatively little immediate attention. A more complete understanding of the clinical picture of myocardial infarction is necessary to provide a basis for decisions concerning therapy. For example, the rationale for the use of thrombolytic agents depends upon improved assumptions concerning the role of thrombosis in myocardial infarction.

The Physiologist and Myocardial Infarction

The committee visited several institutions where there was research activity related to the altered circulation following myocardial infarction. In most instances where there are conventional coronary units, few physiologic observations on the altered circulation were being made except for conventional clinical recording of heart rate and blood pressure. In a small number of centers, more elaborate studies are being undertaken, particularly aimed at the circulatory deterioration (heart failure and shock) which occurs in some patients following acute myocardial infarction. Observations included central venous pressure measured by means of an inlying catheter in the superior vena cava, direct readings of arterial pressure, determination of cardiac output and correlation with chemical factors such as lactate production and blood pH. None of these studies had reached a definitive state. Despite many earlier studies on the hemodynamic consequences of myocardial infarction, fundamental questions of mechanism remain unresolved. Lacking this base, one cannot intelligently approach the problems of drug therapy and other resuscitative maneuvers for such patients. Such studies are complicated by the problems of working with critically ill patients and by the ethical considerations involved. The group of investigators interviewed by the committee did not feel that harm to their patients had occurred. In addition to the studies on patients with overt circulatory failure, there would appear to be the need for studies on less seriously ill patients, in an effort to recognize earlier warning of circulatory deterioration. Such studies would be even more of a problem from an ethical standpoint but would become particularly valuable if more effective means of support of patients with circulatory failure might become available.

There is some difference of opinion regarding the potential value of hemodynamic studies. They would indicate the type of circulatory deficit set off by the myocardial infarction, but they probably would not help in elucidating the basic cause. They might lead to more definitive therapy. It would appear that the most productive units carrying out this sort of study are those with only one or two beds. Such studies are so complicated and time-consuming that large coronary care units cannot undertake them on all patients admitted to their area. A large affiliated unit, however, might serve as a useful reservoir of patients.

There are very few past or current studies of the function and interactions of other body systems which may be important in determining the course of patients with myocardial infarction. Limited studies of pulmonary, renal, cerebral, endocrine and metabolic function which are in progress could be expanded to provide greater insight into the factors which determine the course of the disease and the possible effects of intervention.

The Blood and Myocardial Infarction

Blood-borne factors have been considered important in the development of atherosclerosis. Much has been written regarding the role of cholesterol and other lipids in the development of the atherosclerotic plaque. It is not the purpose of the present report to review these factors in the long-range development of the underlying disease of atherosclerosis. With regard to the more immediate problems of myocardial infarction, it has been suggested by some that changes in blood lipid levels, changes in platelet adhesiveness, and subtle changes in clotting factors may be acute factors in precipitating myocardial infarction. The evidence for any of these changes being primary is not great, but the question should be pursued. Indeed, as noted earlier, there is uncertainty regarding the frequency with which coronary thrombosis occurs in myocardial infarction.

Some studies have shown striking changes in the blood viscosity of patients with myocardial infarction but the importance of these observations is not clear.

The development of thrombolytic agents which can be used in man has engendered considerable interest. The possible use of these agents either to prevent the spread of coronary thrombosis or to lyse a thrombus that has already formed is being studied. A small number of observations along this line have been reported in a preliminary fashion. The National Institutes of Health Program on Thrombolytic Agents has been set up in part to answer the need for further studies in this area. At the present time there is not solid demonstrated evidence indicating the clinical usefulness of these procedures.

The use of anticoagulants in coronary artery disease has received widespread attention during the last two decades. Their use has been predominately in (1) the management of acute myocardial infarction, (2) the long-term use in attempted prevention of new episodes of coronary artery disease, and (3) in, to a limited degree, the treatment of angina pectoris. Although some interest in research in these areas is continuing, the majority of these studies have taken place during the past decade. It is well to point out the fundamental differences in concept in the areas of suggested use. In acute myocardial infarction, the anticoagulants are used primarily to prevent thromboembolic episodes arising from an endocardial thrombus formed near the site of infarction. They also, of course, would be of value in preventing the ill effects of thrombophlebitis of any sort under these circumstances. It has been suggested that it may be possible to prevent the spread of an already-formed coronary thrombosis with myocardial infarction. Reports during recent years have given conflicting results, but none is as enthusiastic as the early large cooperative study sponsored by the American Heart Association in the late 1940s. On analysis at this time, it would appear that the contribution to the mortality rate in acute myocardial infarction by thrombo-embolizatian is small. Therefore, its eradication would not produce large or obvious changes in mortality rate. It is probably for this reason that there has been considerable debate. It is furthermore probably true that more modern methods of management of acute myocardial infarction have lessened the hazard of thromboembolic events. Nevertheless, there is a real hazard of thromboembolism, and anticoagulant therapy would appear to have the potential for limited beneficial effects. New studies and evaluations are being undertaken by the Veterans Administration at this time.

Clinical Pharmacology and Myocardial Infarction

Throughout the nation, about 30 percent of the patients admitted to hospitals with proven myocardial infarction die; it is clear that the problem of treatment is a major one. The prevention of death and the reduction of long-term disability are the obvious goals. In the management of patients with an acute myocardial infarction, there are many therapeutic problems. Of predominate interest at the present time are those related to drugs and mechanical circulatory assistance.

The use of drugs in the treatment of myocardial infarction rests largely on the basis of tradition and empirical evaluation of non-systematic clinical experience.

Relief of pain, sedation and control of anxiety are important in the management of myocardial infarction. Many drugs which are presently used for these purposes are of uncertain benefit and have secondary effects which may be harmful.

Arrhythmia has been found to be much more common than previously suspected. The anti-arrhythmia drugs are being studied in several centers but there are few tightly-designed studies which offer great promise of definitive results. Electrical defibrillation and pacing of the heart have saved many lives, but further studies are needed to establish the optimal conditions for the use of these techniques.

The power failure which results in shock or heart failure is currently treated almost exclusively with drugs, but the high mortality of patients with these syndromes attests to the need for improved use of existing drugs and the development of more effective new drugs.

Several potentially effective interventions should be systematically evaluated. These include precise control of the partial pressure of oxygen in arterial blood and infusion of metabolic substrates and hormones and other agents which influence metabolic patterns of the myocardium.

Assist Devices and Myocardial Infarction

A substantial number of patients with myocardial infarction die of cardiogenic shock. Currently, many of them cannot be resuscitated by any combination of therapy based on known pharmacologic or physiologic techniques. Since the mortality rate for this group is extremely high, considerable interest has been aroused in devising means for mechanically assisting the circulation on either a temporary or permanent basis.

Essentially, two quite different experimental approaches are currently being undertaken by those interested in developing a mechanical solution to this otherwise lethal problem. Some investigators have developed pumping systems (including mechanical valves) on an empirical basis and are testing them both in the laboratory and (in a few instances to date) clinically. Although failure — as signified by death of the patient — has invariably, with a single exception, resulted from this type of intervention, a high level of optimism has characterized these reports. There is no reason to doubt that these developments will continue as the present circulatory support systems are modified and new systems are constructed. An alternative approach has been the search for a clearer understanding of those fundamental considerations at work when blood is pumped artificially through substitute chambers and conduits. Inevitably, this has led to experimental models which evaluate such considerations as sheer stress, pressure ramps (positive and negative), nucleation phenomena, laminar or turbulent flow, and the contribution (adverse and favorable) of wall interactions. Despite obvious complexities inherent in these studies of kinetics, heat and mass transfer, particle technology and biochemical reactions, facts are gradually emerging in response to precisely designed experimentation. Nevertheless, very substantial gaps remain in our rational understanding—mechanistically and chemically—of these events. These gaps are such that, at this time, long-term survival of a dog is not possible when the circulation has had prolonged (several days) and major (more than 50 percent cardiac output) support by a mechanical unit. The combined early and delayed lethal consequences to blood pumping exceed an animal's recuperative powers.

In general, some form of mechanical circulatory support has been sought for thorough use of one of these systems:

a. Diastolic pulsing—augmentation by withdrawal of blood during systole with injection during diastole;

b. Extracorporeal veno-arterial pumping in conjunction with an oxygenator;

c. Left heart bypass by means of:
    1. the venous-transatrial septal puncture technique for cannulation;
    2. the intra- or extracorporeal left atrial systemic arte-

rial circuitry with a gas-driven pump of Dale-
Shuster type. This represents a partial bypass whose
contribution can be regulated on the basis of fluc-
tuating left atrial pressures.

3. an intracorporeal series pump;
4. other pump systems.

d. Improved venous pumping through variations on the
   G-suit.

A byproduct of considerable merit which has arisen from the
complicated analyses involved in solving the problems of
mechanical assistance (or replacement) of the human heart has
been the multi- and interdisciplinary cooperations thereby established. The free flux of intellectual challenges within personnel
from engineering, biometry, chemistry, medicine, radiology and
surgery has provided a variety of stimuli critical to the development of important new ideas. This environment, under the best
of such arrangements, has catalyzed progress in biological problem solving.

Among the very important problems intimately identified
with mechanical pumping of blood is the significant work which
has been done on developing more favorable surfaces to contain
blood. The concept of electrical bonding of heparin to a
graphite benzalkonium surface pioneered thinking in this area
and resulted in a wall (temporarily) superior to all existing artificial boundary layers in the prevention of thrombogenesis in
flowing blood. More recently, investigators have synthesized
polymers in which a chemical bonding of heparin yielded a
reactive surface from which the heparin is not nearly so readily
leached. More important, this surface appears to establish a
dynamic relationship with essential clotting components such
that bleeding and clotting reactions in other parts of the subject
are not abnormal; yet, clots do not form in the tube. The flex-

life and other critical considerations for these materials await further testing. A dacron velour bonded to silastic appears to incorporate in an improved fashion with essential elements from the blood. Almost no precise data, however, are available for analysis of its effects on flowing blood.

Cardiac Revascularization.

Cardiac revascularization has two aspects: (1) supplying the heart by non-coronary vessels, and (2) modification of the situation so that muscle survives long enough for new channels to develop from existing coronary arteries. This is, in effect, aiding the natural revascularization process. Encouraging progress is being made in both fields.

Recent demonstrations at several cardiovascular centers of the long-term patency of internal mammary arterial implants into the myocardium have renewed widespread interest in revascularization procedures. In fact, at least a half-dozen different operations designed to augment the cardiac blood supply are currently under laboratory and/or clinical testing. Subjective reports of postoperative improvement are of limited value. Unfortunately, almost no reasonably precise quantitative measure is available to assess the accomplishment of the implantation procedures in terms of unquestionably "proving" that life-saving protection against coronary death has been achieved. In fact, few studies have even measured alterations in substrate utilization by the myocardium before and after vascular augmentation of the normal or the ischemic myocardium. Studies of myocardial lactate extraction and production before and after attempts at myocardial revascularization revealed a conversion from anaerobic to aerobic metabolism in some persons. However, methods for quantitating the volume of new blood available for myocardial metabolism have generally been unsatisfactory. This difficulty has not been suitably met through various angiographic techniques, comparison of arterial and coronary sinus differences, or use of a variety of isotopic methods designed to calculate myocardial flow. Flowmeters on the implant vessel likewise fail to identify the volume of new blood reaching the cellular level. On the positive side, recent work has clearly demonstrated the equivalent capacity of the non-ischemic heart to develop collateral communications with the transplanted vessel. Thus, at least this aspect of certain experimental models has now been clarified. True, qualitative impressions about revascularization can be secured from some studies of late filling of proximally-obstructed coronary branches.

The critical importance of such collateral flow is clearly implied in the studies of survival after coronary obstruction. Investigators have demonstrated statistically greater survival rates in dogs subjected to ligation of the anterior descending coronary artery (distal to the lateral ventricular branch) when the tie-off is followed by a period of two hours of extracorporeal counter pulsation (together with heparinization). Specifically, in those animals so treated, (1) the incidence of early deaths after ligation was lower, and (2) the coronary collateral arborization was demonstrably superior and retrograde filling of the proximal branches up to the site of ligation was regularly more complete. For these several reasons, therefore, the search for increasingly effective revascularization procedures should continue.

Rehabilitation and Myocardial Infarction

Rehabilitation is properly viewed as an integral part of the therapy of myocardial infarction. There is little critical information concerning optimal convalescent care of the patient with myocardial infarction, and there is consequently little basis for judging the potential salvage to be realized from improved techniques of rehabilitation. The traditional program of prolonged rest and restriction of activity is intended to minimize the work of the heart during the period of several months required for full development of collateral circulation in the myocardium. It is not certain that this rationale is valid or pertinent, or what specific rest-activity program is best. There is no evidence that those who reject parts of the prescribed programs have a different incidence of complications. The effect of extreme variation from the traditional programs may reasonably be studied in animals, while critical analysis of current experience in man, coupled with clinical experiments within the range of accepted practice or involving more modest departure from accepted practice, may be useful in developing more effective programs of rehabilitation.

Research Potential of Myocardial Infarction Study Centers

While numerous studies fundamental to the better understanding and more effective treatment of myocardial infarction can be conducted in the laboratory, the ultimate test of the applicability of such observations and the assessment of proposed therapy must be performed on patients. There was general agreement that the presence of a coronary care unit increases the likelihood of staff becoming involved in clinical research. It was regarded as a very desirable asset but not an obligatory facility for the conduct of clinical investigation of myocardial infarction.

Optimal medical care for the patient with myocardial infarction can be rendered most efficiently in a cardiac care unit which brings together patients with myocardial infarction in an environment of specialized monitoring and therapeutic devices, and an adequate and specially-trained staff. A similar environment is desirable for most clinical investigations on myocardial infarction.

The experience at several centers has demonstrated that valuable investigation can be conducted in such facilities and that the patients being studied receive superior clinical care. The doctors in charge of these units believe that the chances of recovery are increased when the patients are in the research units.

To date, research in the cardiac care unit has been directed more at a description of the natural course of myocardial infarction than at the careful evaluation of therapeutic interventions. Several centers, however, are now initiating programs to assess the efficacy of anti-arrhythmic and other pharmacologic agents and mechanical devices.

Most studies have depended upon electrocardiographic monitoring, indirect hemodynamic measurements, and in vitro chemical determinations. Computer and instrumentation development have been the focus of some laboratories. Attention is currently shifting to direct hemodynamic measurements, including prolonged pulmonary artery pressure measurement and direct intra-arterial pressure determinations and cardiac output measurement by indicator dilution techniques. Physicians engaged in pioneering studies in at least three centers, with an accumulated experience of over 200 patients, have demonstrated to their own satisfaction that these measurements can be performed continuously for 24 to 48 hours without adverse effect.

More extensive clinical investigation of the patient acutely ill with myocardial infarction has been limited by a number of factors:

1. The proper caution for conducting studies which might interfere with ordinary clinical care or which might in themselves have a deleterious effect on the patient.
2. The difficulties of following a research protocol while investigating a multifaceted and rapidly changing illness associated with a relatively high mortality.

3. The expense of establishing and running a clinical research unit, particularly with the difficulties of obtaining research funding for an operation so intimately related to patient care.
4. The need for around-the-clock staffing by specially trained technicians and nurses, as well as investigators.
5. The limited applicability of existing instrumentation and techniques to this clinical setting.
6. The problems of handling and analyzing continuously accumulating data.

It is evident that each of these factors retarding research in the coronary care unit can be ameliorated by a properly focused program and by the accumulation of clinical experience.

Certain policies and facilities seem particularly desirable for a research-focused coronary care unit, perhaps better termed a Myocardial Infarction Study Center (MISC).

The central role of cardiology in such a center is evident but, in general, a well-integrated, multidisciplinary research program, which may include close ties to non-clinical laboratories, will be of greatest value. Carefully integrated, comprehensive studies on relatively few patients will in many instances be more desirable than limited studies in larger numbers of patients. Some investigations will focus on a precise characterization of the natural course of the acute illness while others will deal primarily with the development or assessment of therapeutic interventions.

All patients in the MISC should be study patients and under full control of the director; thus, additional coronary care facilities should exist for patients not entering the study and for patients after the study period. Patients who have been the subjects of detailed, comprehensive study during the course of their acute illness should, whenever possible, be subjects for study during rehabilitation and long-term follow-up. The number of patients available for study and the scope of investigations should be sufficiently great to permit efficient utilization of the facility and its staff.

Physical facilities should include quiet, single rooms large enough for bringing in research apparatus. Proximity to other facilities, such as the coronary care unit, fluoroscopy, operating rooms and special chemistry laboratories, may be particularly important. Instrumentation should include apparatus for measuring pertinent electrical, hemodynamic, biochemical and other parameters with minimal constraints upon the patients. The system must integrate transducers, signal processors, display and alarm devices and apparatus for data storage, retrieval, analysis and computation. Some uniformity in measurement and data storage techniques must exist among the MISC's to permit comparison of data, possible analysis of data at a single facility, and upgrading of all MISC instrumentation systems as new developments occur.

Staffing of the MISC's must include experienced doctors who are also expert clinical investigators of the highest caliber. Nurses and technicians must be specially trained, and their number must take into account the greater demands of research protocols.

Funding must be adequate for establishing the research facility and for paying operational costs above routine patient care; commitments must be sufficiently long-term to permit long-range staffing.

Research in the myocardial infarction study center may be expected to have a number of beneficial results.

The better description of the natural course of myocardial infarction, with correlation of the pathophysiology of different organ systems, will lead to a better understanding of the illness and ultimately to its more effective therapy. The identification of the most significant and sensitive parameters for prognostic and monitoring purposes will facilitate research in the MISC; more importantly, it will lead to better patient care in all coronary care units by permitting recognition of patients requiring particular attention and by permitting practical monitoring techniques based on only a limited number of parameters.

The Myocardial Infarction Study Centers will permit the development of more effective therapeutic techniques. The results of previous studies in myocardial infarction have been severely jeopardized by failure to separate patients into homogeneous subgroups. The controlled environment and specialized facilities of the Myocardial Infarction Study Centers will permit the more precise characterization of individual patients and their classification into subgroups, thereby providing more clear-cut results from studies on fewer patients. The study centers will make possible the study of a wider range of therapeutic interventions than was heretofore possible. The more careful and complete study of interventions will permit a better assessment of both the value and the side effects of proposed therapy; it will permit the assessment of therapy by precise endpoints other than crude mortality, thereby clarifying the effects of therapy by investigations on fewer patients. A step-by-step reduction of mortality may result from identifying interventions which individually may have only a small effect upon mortality. The more precise recognition of shortcomings of proposed therapy will permit the more ready development of new and successful therapeutic techniques. Furthermore, current regimens for the treatment of myocardial infarction became firmly established before any critical quantitative study of their effects and side effects was possible; thus careful study and appraisal of what is already accepted therapy is an important topic for investigation.

The improvement in patient salvage brought about by the development of resuscitation techniques and continuous patient monitoring, has demonstrated that the course of myocardial infarction can be altered favorably, and it has created a climate highly favorable for clinical research. Further clinical investigation on myocardial infarction is expected to yield a still better understanding of the illness and, more importantly, its more effective treatment.

The existing or projected coronary care units represent a good base for an expanded research program. The establishment of a number of clinical myocardial infarction research centers is a necessary part of the myocardial infarction program.

Instrumentation Needs of Myocardial Infarction Study Centers

The scientists interviewed were in general agreement that more effective instrumentation would significantly enhance clinical research on myocardial infarction.

It is the assessment of the committee that instrumentation in the myocardial infarction study center must provide both the data for patient care and for the research protocol. In addition, some forms of therapy under investigation may have a major instrumentation component.

Presently, most coronary care units have instrumentation monitoring systems centered on the electrocardiogram. Some units are moving to direct hemodynamic measurements and pioneering research groups have brought other apparatus into the research coronary care unit for metabolic, pulmonary and renal function measurement. Most systems represent a custom assembly of off-the-shelf transducers, recorders, display and alarm devices; some groups have utilized computers; and a few have made research in instrumentation for the acutely ill patient a major focus of their attention.

Present-day apparatus and techniques are not optimal for clinical investigation, and foreseeable improvements in instrumentation and data handling would significantly enhance the scope, the safety, and quality of clinical research.

The Myocardial Infarction Program should foster the development of instrumentation and techniques to meet the needs of its clinical research program. It should also foster policies which will ensure the comparability of data obtained in the various centers within the program. Toward this latter goal, it should establish detailed specifications for much of the instrumentation used in these centers and conformity to these standards should be maintained.

To meet the needs of clinical research, the program should foster the development of an integrated instrumentation system which imposes minimum restraint and hazard to the patient but which provides maximum data. The system should be simple to operate and much of its functioning should be automatic. It should make data available immediately, both for patient care and for research. It should also provide apparatus for data storage, retrieval, correlation and analysis. The system should include sensors and transducers, signal processors and alarm devices, and apparatus for recording, display, rapid recall, analysis and computation. The input to the system might include not only physiological and biochemical parameters under study, but also the therapy in progress, measurements of the environment, and a record of non-instrumental observations. The output of the system should include display and monitoring devices and permanent research records as well as immediately available clinical records of the measured factors and certain derived functions. These records would be valuable both for immediate patient care and for the research protocol. The system should be developed to meet the requirements common to most centers within the program, but it should have the flexibility to accommodate the specialized needs of individual centers, and it should be compatible with foreseeable instrumentation needs and developments.

This instrumentation program can be considered to have

four subprograms:

1. The analysis of systems needs and the development of an integrated instrumentation system to be available within one year. This system should primarily utilize off-the-shelf hardware and techniques, but it should be compatible with foreseeable instrumentation needs and developments.

2. The development of those instrumentation and data—handling techniques which cannot be brought to fruition so quickly, but which are clearly foreseeable and represent step-by-step developments of currently available apparatus and techniques.

3. Fostering the developments of techniques in instrumentation so different and far-reaching as to be dependent upon break-throughs rather than clearly predictable development.

4. The development of instrumentation primarily of a therapeutic nature.

The effective integration of these multiple functions for the numerous factors under study is a significant task and it is a valuable goal. The analysis of instrumentation system needs and the development of such a system should be an early step in the myocardial infarction program.

Research Potential of Animal Models of Myocardial Infarction

It is generally agreed that moral, ethical and practical restraints limit the range of investigations of patients with myocardial infarction and, in many instances, cause a compromise in the quality of experimental design. One possible means of developing information not otherwise available is the use of animal models of the human disease. There is not uniformity of judgment concerning the potential value of such models. One view is that since ultimate answers must come from studies of man, animal studies should not have a major place in a myocardial infarction research program.

An alternate judgment holds that in many aspects of current and potential management of myocardial infarction and in understanding of the disease, there is need for experiments which cannot be done in man. These experiments would probably include the study of: (1) factors which precipitate myocardial infarction; (2) metabolism of ischemic myocardium; (3) pharmacologic interventions; and (4) surgical interventions. The concensus favors the judgment that development and availability of appropriate animal models of myocardial infarction would offer important opportunities to improve understanding and management of myocardial infarction.

The necessary characteristics of potential animal models are not well established. For some purposes, acute surgically-induced infarction in previously healthy animals may be sufficient; other studies may require animals with previously injured and scarred myocardium or animals with their coronary circulation compromised by gradually developing obstructing lesions. Models are available with varying degrees of similarity to human disease. The highest degree of similarity is possibly the primate with coronary atherosclerosis. There is reason to believe that such animals could be produced in substantial numbers, but the real advantages of this expensive model are not certain.

Reaction of Our Colleagues to the Program of Increasing the Research Effort in the Therapy of Acute Myocardial Infarction

Myocardial infarction is an event in the course of a generalized disease of blood vessels. The treatment of acute myocardial infarction will not prevent the progression of atherosclerosis. Is there justification for a program designed to support a more intensive effort at understanding and treatment of this episode in the course of a progressive process?

Our colleagues reacted to the above formulation of the problem in many ways. The more pessimistic said that prevention of atherosclerosis should be the ultimate goal, and that our resources should be devoted to its prevention rather than to the treatment of its complications. The more optimistic believed that an intensive effort to increase immediate survival from acute myocardial infarction would yield fruitful results and was mandatory. The following paragraph summarizes the viewpoint of most of the people whom we interviewed.

While a solution to the problem of atherosclerosis would be of greater benefit than simply the more effective treatment of myocardial infarction, the latter was nevertheless felt to be a realistic and important goal.

The more effective treatment of myocardial infarction deserves the highest priority for targeted research for several reasons:

1. the major importance of myocardial infarction as a cause of death and disability in thecommunity;
2. sufficient fundamental knowledge, new ideas, research techniques, committed and trained investigators and funds can be brought to bear upon the problem to yield significant results; and
3. additional research monies will bring new personnel and ideas into this field.

The majority of the medical community believes that money invested in research without central coordination and a defined developmental goal eventually pays the greatest dividends and is the most likely source of important major new concepts.

Accordingly, no one is enthusiastic about a new program centered on reducing the mortality of myocardial infarction at the expense of the existing grant-in-aid programs. There is no doubt that dollars invested in a program for research with the objective of improved treatment of myocardial infarction can carry us a certain distance toward the goal of reducing the mortality from myocardial infarction. Existing concepts, however, do not in fact offer the prospect of eliminating myocardial infarction as a major cause of death. Support for pertinent undirected research, the primary source of new ideas, should not be compromised.

There is the realistic fear that a program of research in myocardial infarction may become part of the funding pattern of certain institutions and that research positions in this program may be filled at the expense of more gifted investigators who are not interested in the myocardial infarction program. Our colleagues repeatedly advise us of the necessity for effective control of the quality of personnel and research.

The committee believes that well-designed, goal-directed research should properly be a part of our total research effort on myocardial infarction. It should supplement but never replace non-directed research.

Ethical Considerations Concerning Clinical Research on Myocardial Infarction

There have not been extensive clinical studies of myocardial infarction in the past, in part because the prospect of benefit to the patient did not seem sufficient to justify the risks of the potential research projects. With the development of improved techniques of treatment, new kinds of patient-care facilities and advances in research techniques and experiences, the risks of certain kinds of research are being defined and reduced and, accordingly, some of the ethical constraints on clinical research on patients with myocardial infarction are being relieved. For this reason, ethical limitations on research can be expected to change continuously, both in the country at large and in individual research units.

It is clear that valuable observations in the natural history and course of the disease can be made by systematic collection and analysis of data which is now collected for patient care. Such studies involve no change in patient care whatsoever and therefore pose no unusual ethical problem. Recording of usual clinical data with the information from more extensive electrocardiographic monitoring, combined with usual clinical and laboratory measurements, would establish tighter subgroups of the illness which would serve as a better base for prognosis and for additional research. Everyone agreed that electrocardiographic monitoring is desirable. Most physicians are willing to make serial measurements on all patients which do not involve needles or catheters.

There is a group of patients in whom the results of the illness are so catastrophic that ethical considerations force collection of extensive data which, for optimal patient care, should be of research quality. For example, everyone agrees that there is a group of patients with circulatory failure who do not respond quickly to medical management and that in these patients the mortality is in excess of 70 percent. In these patients, extensive clinical research is clearly indicated, and the usual measurements made by a sophisticated shock team are desirable.

The science of care of the critically ill patient is not rigorously developed. For this reason, there are many times when "therapeutic trials" are attempted and when, in the judgment of the physician, it is not in the best interest of the patient to discuss the implications of the trial. While the analysis of data from such therapeutic trials does in fact constitute research, the intervention and the observations are made for the purpose of patient care, and the appropriate ethical considerations are those which apply to the practice of medicine.

There is a spectrum of opinions on the desirability of introducing research protocols into a coronary care unit. Some physicians fear that research interests would interfere with patient care; others believe that research protocols would sharpen patient care. In some medical centers, the staff has demonstrated to their own satisfaction that patient care has already been improved by quantitative measurement in coronary care units. These centers would welcome the opportunity to increase their research activities on patients.

It is repeatedly emphasized that what is ethical for one physician is not ethical for another. A physician who strongly believes that anti-arrhythmic drugs are important in reducing mortality cannot ethically randomize his patients into a treated and non-treated series. A physician who believes that the drugs selected are neither useful nor harmful can ethically randomize the patients. It is generally agreed that many problems raised by clinical research must be taken to the animal laboratory before additional clinical research is either ethical or desirable.

In summary, the committee believes that, while ethical considerations will impose restraints on research on myocardial infarction and while in some cases, new experimental designs will have to be developed to meet ethical criteria, a broad range of important research problems can be addressed within current and projected ethical standards.

Reactions of the Committee

Administration of a Myocardial Infarction Program

The scientific community recognizes that acute myocardial

infarction is a major cause of death and agrees that one of the goals of the National Heart Institute should be to reduce the mortality of acute myocardial infarction.

The problem is a difficult one to attack because it is many-faceted, and there is no single solution which will be suitable to all patients. It involves research centered around patients with a high immediate mortality and the necessity for having the combination of the best clinical care and around-the-clock research teams. It involves the use of expensive space for patients and scientists in the most crowded and expensive portions of our medical centers. The problems cannot be solved by physicians and surgeons alone. Suitable physical and social structures have to be devised which can tap the best scientific brains in the universities. In the opinion of the committee, new administrative devices within the NHI and new relations between the scientific community and the NHI will have to be developed if one wishes to move more rapidly toward the goal of a reduction in mortality from acute myocardial infarction.

Methods must be devised which can effectively mobilize the resources of government to make it possible for universities to mount programs involving research in patients with acute illness. The resources needed are:

1. clinical staff and scientists from the key disciplines related to the problem;
2. support for patients both during the acute studies and for those patients whose life is prolonged non-productively because of the research;
3. support for around-the-clock clinical staff and for paramedical staff;
4. training programs for paramedical staff; and
5. creation of space for scientists related to the program.

We need to devise mechanisms where we can identify that

portion of the community which is both capable and willing to direct its efforts toward the goal of a reduction in the mortality of acute myocardial infarction. These persons might apply for funds under the review of a continuing advisory group responsible for the scientific excellence of the programs. One of the requirements for submitting an application might be the acceptance of the goal of reducing the mortality from acute myocardial infarction. The principal investigators under this program would agree to meet three times a year to review their own progress and to identify those areas where the NHI could profitably stimulate work which might shorten the time to reach the agreed goal. Once each year the principal investigators and NHI staff might review the total program and recommend to the advisory group those programs no longer relevant to the goal be supported elsewhere or discontinued. Every five years the special advisory group might review the programs to see that they remain goal-directed.

The NHI staff will have the role of devising effective, coordinated programs which will allow the scientists, both extramural and intramural, the opportunity for most effective work. It cannot assume the role of principal scientist contracting with others for needed work. The fear that the NHI may not recognize this limitation is one of the reasons why the academic community prefers grants to contracts.

In summary, the committee recommends that new types of flexible support be established to allow more direct progress toward an accepted NHI goal. It knows that funding on a broad front to attack the problem of acute myocardial infarction in depth will involve some duplication and some wandering from the goal, but it believes that substantial progress toward the goal can be achieved. It believes that a narrow program directed only toward immediately identifiable, useful clinical points will not achieve the goal.

Promising Elements of a Myocardial Infarction Program

Recent research efforts have already resulted in improvement in patient care. (1) The combination of external massage, assisted respiration and defibrillation have been effective in saving lives of individual patients with acute myocardial infarction. Some of these patients are now living useful and effective lives. For the first time in the last 20 years, all medical centers are interested in more aggressive care of patients with myocardial infarction. (2) The catheter pacing of patients with acute myocardial infarction has saved individual lives. (3) Acute myocardial infarction has always had a high mortality and the survivors have had a high morbidity. This morbidity was in part dependent on the damage to the heart but, in considerable part, dependent on the reaction of the patient, family, friends and community to the acute heart attack. All observers agree that intelligent emotional and physical rehabilitation programs are effective in reducing morbidity. (4) The few investigators using electrocardiographic and hemodynamic monitoring as a guide to drug, fluid and electrolyte therapy all believe they prevent deaths from acute Infarction. They emphasize that drugs may be used most effectively when monitoring is effective. There is some evidence that ventricular fibrillation may be prevented by drug therapy.

Assisted circulation offers the hope of increasing the survival rate of those patients in whom death results from muscle failure. This is an educated guess, but the development of assist devices which can remain in place for long periods of time is accepted as a realistic goal. There is more doubt about the usefulness of short-time support systems after the heart is massively infarcted. Will enough recovery be possible to sustain a useful existence? This matter can be settled only by appropriate clinical observations.

Adequate revascularization of the heart may be possible. More time and effort can be profitably spent on research to devise methods to salvage the patient with massive infarction if the long-term prognosis can be improved. Revascularization of the heart offers at present our best chance for modifying the natural history of coronary atherosclerosis. Supplying the heart with more blood has a better statistical chance of improving overall mortality of atherosclerosis than does revascularization of any other part of the body.

The high mortality in coronary artery disease cannot be reduced by hospital care alone, as many patients die before they reach the doctor. Prospective studies can identify the population most likely to have a myocardial infarction. Sample electrocardiographic monitoring of this population may define the portion of this infarct-prone population which is at greatest risk from sudden death. Factors which cause the development of infarction and those which, in the presence of coronary arterial disease cause fatal arrhythmia without infarction, may be identified and better methods of management may be defined.

Broadened and extended clinical research can afford significant new opportunities for understanding the biologic phenomenon of myocardial infarction. It can provide for a needed critical and systematic assessment of current therapy as a basis for improved utilization of interventions which are now available, and it can provide a further stimulus for the development of new agents along with a means for rapid and discriminating evaluation of these agents.

Clinical research on patients with myocardial infarction would have a rich series of secondary gains.

The development of facilities, techniques and instrumentation for studying patients with myocardial infarction are equally applicable to the study of patients acutely ill with other diseases. The more complete observations on these patients will provide new insight into basic pathophysiology, which will likely be applicable to the understanding and treatment of other disease.

A broad base of non-clinical research and development can sustain and advance the clinical research of a myocardial infarction program. This work will range from instrument development through fundamental but relevant biology. In large measure, clinical elements of the program must draw on activities of the general scientific community for this support, but additional support for specific efforts is needed.

The committee concludes that, at this point in time, the National Heart Institute can, with profit, direct a portion of its research effort toward creating a program aimed at improving the treatment of acute myocardial infarction.

Summary and Recommendations

This committee appointed by the late Dr. Robert Grant has surveyed the scientific community to (1) determine the present status of our knowledge of myocardial infarction and its treatment; (2) make a judgment as to whether it is reasonable for the National Heart Institute to make as one of its immediate research goals the solution of identifiable problems which will lead to the improved therapy of this illness; and (3) determine the potential usefulness of coronary care units as a research base for an intensified research effort to improve the treatment of acute myocardial infarction.

We identified no single approach to the problem of improving the treatment of patients with acute myocardial infarction. We did identify a number of people and institutions who were interested in intensifying their work on problems relating to the problem of acute myocardial infarction. In each instance, the research workers emphasized the complexity of the problem and the necessity for approaching the problem from many angles.

They had the usual needs for space, research scientists and equipment. In addition, they needed facilities and training programs for around-the-clock operation of a clinical research unit, housing patients with an acute illness and a high mortality. They needed access to equipment capable of handling large masses of data generated by around-the-clock observations. They needed to have many measurements which could be repeated at frequent intervals and facilities for assembling data from many areas to supply the needed information for rapid decision-making.

The committee was given supporting data which indicate that much can be accomplished if the research effort is both broad and intensive, and that coronary care units offer an attractive place to center much of the program. In general, these units are structured for patient care, and the clinical research programs must be built in. Ideally, the unit should have strong clinical leadership in cardiology, with good support from such disciplines as surgery, biochemistry, radiology, and hematology. Active related programs in the animal laboratory, in bioengineering and in data processing would add greatly to the research capabilities of the coronary care unit.

The committee found no coronary care unit which had all these components, but many had a number of them already present and there was interest in adding others. Some active programs ready for expansion do not have coronary care units.

The committee recommends that the National Heart Institute should expand its research program in the area of acute myocardial infarction. The program will require the addition of research capabilities to existing coronary care units and a program to train paramedical personnel to operate effectively in these research areas. It will require the addition of scientists from many disciplines with supporting equipment and supplies, and it will require animal laboratories, animal models of myocardial infarction and data processing units.

New relationships will have to be worked out between the scientific community and the National Heart Institute staff if the goal of improved treatment is to be met within the next five to 10 years. The National Heart Institute staff will have to devise ways to bring effective financing to support the complex mixture of clinical science, clinical care, basic science and bioengineering needed in this program. It will have to develop better methods for communications so that new ideas are not stifled but that the goal of better therapy is not lost. It will have to take more leadership in the development of instrumentation and centralized data processing. The scientific community taking part in this program must be willing to discipline itself to insure progress toward the agreed goal. It must pool its data, accept common standards for measurement, and take part in the conferences and symposia which will be necessary to move toward the agreed goal.

The grants system, in its present form, has not nurtured this type of interaction between grantees or between grantees and the National Heart Institute. The usual collaborative programs seem unsuited for a problem which must be attacked by multiple approaches and at various levels. The traditional contract programs seem unduly restrictive for the best interests of a myocardial infarction program. The committee therefore recommends that the National Heart Institute and the scientific community explore new administrative devices to accomplish the objectives recommended in this report.